Hospice Programs and Public Policy

Edited by Paul R. Torrens, M.D., M.P.H.

American Hospital Publishing, Inc.,
a wholly owned subsidiary
of the American Hospital Association

The views expressed in this book are those of Paul R. Torrens
and other contributing authors.

Library of Congress Cataloging in Publication Data
Main entry under title:

Hospice programs and public policy.

  Includes bibliographies.
  1. Hospices (Terminal care) — Addresses, essays,
lectures. 2. Hospice care — Addresses, essays, lectures.
3. Medical ethics — Addresses, essays, lectures.
I. Torrens, Paul R.
R726.8.H672 1984   362.1'75   84-21642
ISBN 0-939450-48-8

Catalog no. 193100

©1985 by American Hospital Publishing, Inc.,
a wholly owned subsidiary of the American Hospital Association.

AHA is a service mark of the American Hospital Association
used under license by American Hospital Publishing, Inc.

Printed in the U.S.A.

2M-11/84-0055

Beryl Dwight, Editor
Gretchen Messer, Production Coordinator
Marjorie E. Weissman, Manager, Book Editorial
Dorothy Saxner, Vice-President, Books

*It is not right that death
should be such a lonely
technological event.*

——Paul Beeson

Contents

Part 1   History and Background of Hospice Programs
         in the United States

Chapter 1   Development of Special Care Programs for the Dying:
             Paul R. Torrens, M.D., M.P.H.

Chapter 2
             Paul R. Torrens, M.D., M.P.H.

Chapter 3
             Paul R. Torrens, M.D., M.P.H.

Part 2   Issues in Hospice Care in the United States

Chapter 4
             Paul R. Torrens, M.D., M.P.H.

List of Figures

List of Tables

Acknowledgments

It is difficult to acknowledge all of the individuals and organizations, all of the experiences and insights, that have made this book possible, because so many people and so many organizations have contributed to its content.

First in time, my friends and colleagues in the Veterans Administration — both in Washington, DC, and in the Wadsworth Veterans Administration Hospital in Los Angeles — provided the specific experience for me of seeing one hospice program develop and grow. Ed O'Neill, Joe Mason, Earl Gordon, Jack Chase, Bill Anderson, Paul Haber, Sharon Garrett, Ed Olsen, Robert Krasnow, Jeff Wales, and Bob Kane have all been important in the development of the palliative care program at Wadsworth and in the growth of my learning.

The Pan American Health Organization provided me with a World Health Organization Traveling Fellowship in 1979, which made it possible for me to review at first hand the development of hospice programs in England, Scotland, and Wales.

In the British Isles, the welcome and support of colleagues was beyond expectation. Cicely Saunders, Tom West, and Dorothy Summers at St. Christopher's, Richard Hillyer in Southampton, Ronald Fischer in Christchurch, Pru Clench in Bath, Eric Wilkes in Sheffield, Richard Lamerton at St. Joseph's in Hackney, and Derreck Doyle in Edinburgh were particularly helpful with specific programs, and Paul Sturgess of the Marie Curie Memorial Foundation, Colonel Garnett of the National Society for Cancer Relief, and Gillian Ford of the Department of Health and Social Security all provided me with a view of the broad issues of hospice care in England. As always, Ian Munro and Robyn Fox of *Lancet* and George Godber, former chief medical officer for the National Health Service, provided me with thoughtful reflections on all that I was learning.

In Canada, Barbara McCutcheon, Dorothy Ley, Darlene Flett, and Elma Heidemann of the Palliative Care Foundation of Canada were most helpful in providing information and insights about the current status of hospice programs in that country.

Closer to home, I am greatly indebted to my colleagues who have agreed to write chapters in this book and who have generously contributed their time and insights to help shape its broad outlines. They have given of themselves and their talents far beyond the call of duty, and I am very grateful. I can only hope that the quality of the final product is just recompense for their efforts on its behalf.

In a very practical way, Annette Lefcourt, Marylyn Taber, Jean Sellen, and Andrea Larson have helped organize my life so that it was possible to have the time and energy to devote to this work. Mary Hunter and her colleagues in the word processing center at the University of California at Los Angeles have been remarkably efficient in taking my draft materials and turning them into finished manuscript copies in record time and without complaint. At the American Hospital Association, Ellen Pryga of the Division of Health Policy and Financing read and carefully critiqued the manuscript, and at American Hospital Publishing, Inc., Beryl Dwight has been that most valued of colleagues — a supportive and patient editor.

Finally, to the hospice patients and their families everywhere, from whom I have learned the most important lessons about hospice care, I extend my greatest thanks. It is to your memory that this book is dedicated.

Paul R. Torrens

Contributors

Linda Aiken, Ph.D., a registered nurse, is vice-president for research at the Robert Wood Johnson Foundation in Princeton, New Jersey, and is chairman of the medical sociology section of the American Sociological Association. She has a doctorate in sociology from the University of Texas at Austin and has done postdoctoral work in medical sociology at the University of Wisconsin.

John D. Blum, J.D., M.S., is associate professor of health planning and administration at Pennsylvania State University, University Park. A lawyer with additional graduate education in health services administration, he is interested in health law and regulation on both the state and federal level. He has been connected with programs for the care of the dying since 1978, when he first became associated with Omega, a freestanding community-based, volunteer-staffed program in Cambridge, Massachusetts. More recently, he has been associated with the hospice program of the Centre County Home Health Agency in Bellefonte, Pennsylvania.

Mary Cummings, Dr.P.H., while director of research for the Kaiser-Permanente Medical Care Program, Southern California Region, Los Angeles, was one of the initiators of its hospice program and eventually served as the director of evaluation for that program. She also coordinated a major evaluation, funded by the National Cancer Institute, of three hospice demonstration programs, including a study of costs. For three years, she served as chairman of the evaluation and research committee for the National Hospice Organization.

David J. English, D.P.A., is president of the Center for the Aging of the Greater Southeast Community Hospital Foundation, Washington, DC. From 1977 to 1981, he was president of ELM Services, Inc., a health planning and consulting firm, and was also executive director of the ELM Institute, a not-for-profit research and educational institute. While associated with ELM, he conducted a number of major hospice-related consulting and research projects and was the author of a number of hospice-related planning and management monographs.

Joanne Lynn, M.D., M.A., works predominantly with terminally ill and elderly patients in the Division of Geriatric Medicine in the Department of Health Care Sciences at the George Washington University Medical Center, Washington, DC. She is attending physician for the inpatient hospice at the Washington Home. She was the assistant director for medical studies for the President's Commission for the Study of Ethical Problems in Medicine and Biomedical and Behavioral Research and led the drafting of the commission's report *Deciding to Forego Life-Sustaining Treatment*.

Martita Marx, Dr.P.H., was a senior program officer at the Robert Wood Johnson Foundation in Princeton, New Jersey, at the time of the writing of the article included in this volume as chapter 12. At the foundation, she had the responsibility for coordinating the foundation's participation in the major, 26-site research study of the financing of hospice care under Medicare, sponsored by the Robert Wood Johnson Foundation, the John Hartford Foundation, and the U.S. Health Care Financing Administration.

Marian Osterweis, Ph.D., is a medical sociologist who is currently director of a study on the health consequences of bereavement for the Institute of Medicine, National Academy of Sciences, Washington, DC. Previously, she was a member of the faculty of the Department of Community and Family Medicine at Georgetown University School of Medicine for 10 years and was a staff member of the President's Commission for the Study of Ethical Problems in Medicine and Biomedical and Behavioral Research. For that commission, she was primarily responsible for the report *Making Health Care Decisions: The Ethical and Legal Implications of Informed Consent in the Patient-Practitioner Relationship*. She has been associated with hospice programs for six years as a member of the planning committee for an inpatient hospice unit in a nursing home, as a hospice evaluator, and as a consultant to several hospice programs.

Dennis A. Robbins, Ph.D., M.P.H., is director of the graduate program in health administration at Salve Regina College, Newport, Rhode Island. A former fellow of the National Fund for Medical Education at the Kennedy Interfaculty Program in Medical Ethics at Harvard University, his professional interests combine ethics, law, and health services policy. A member of the International Work Group on Death, Dying, and

Bereavement, he is the coeditor of *Ethical Dimensions of Clinical Medicine* (1981) and the author of *Legal and Ethical Issues in Cancer Care in the United States* (1983). Dr. Robbins was the executive vice-president of the Hospice of Lower Cape Fear in Wilmington, North Carolina, from 1979 to 1980.

Claire Tehan, M.A., has been the hospice program director for the Hospital Home Health Care Agency in Torrance, California since 1978. Prior to that, she was the hospice program coordinator for the University of Rochester Cancer Center for two years. She has served on the board of directors of the National Hospice Organization since 1980 and was the vice-president in 1981-1982. She has served on the board of directors of the Southern California Hospice Association since 1979 and was vice-president (1979-1980) and president (1980-1981) of that organization. She has served on the National Hospice Organization committee on standards and accreditation since 1980 and has also served on the hospice advisory committee of the Joint Commission on Accreditation of Hospitals since 1981.

Paul Torrens, M.D., M.P.H., is professor of health services administration at the University of California at Los Angeles School of Public Health and has long been interested in the overall functioning of the American health care system and the public policy issues that affect it. He was the recipient of a World Health Organization traveling fellowship in 1979 to study hospice programs in England, Scotland, and Wales, and was one of the initiators of the Palliative Care Unit at the Wadsworth Veterans Administration Hospital in Los Angeles. He currently serves as the chairman of the advisory committee for that unit and is also a member of the board of directors of the Hospice Organization of Southern California.

Jeffrey Wales, Ph.D., is a medical sociologist who was the project director for the University of California at Los Angeles Hospice Evaluation Study at the Wadsworth Veterans Administration Hospital. An assistant professor in the School of Public Health at UCLA, he was previously an assistant professor of gerontology and sociology at the University of Southern California. His major area of professional interest is the application of new research and evaluation techniques to health and welfare programs.

Dottie C. Wilson is the director of the Palliative Care Center, St. Mary's Hospital for Children, Bayside, New York. From 1974 to 1978, she was the administrator of the Palliative Care Service of the Royal Victoria Hospital in Montreal, and from 1978 until she assumed her present position in 1981, she was the manager of hospice activities for the ELM Institute and the director of hospice development and technical assistance for ELM Services, Inc., both in Rockville, Maryland.

Introduction

In 1951, the Marie Curie Memorial Foundation in England conducted a national survey on the care of cancer patients who were nursed at home and arrived at some important conclusions. "It is obvious to us that considerable hardship exists in the case of many families who are taking care of one member with cancer at home. In addition to providing skilled nursing treatment for the patient, the provision of residential homes would save much mental suffering, stress, and strain for the patients and the relatives. Beds in the hospitals might also be freed."[1]

When the report was published, Cicely Saunders was just entering medical school at St. Thomas's Hospital Medical School in London, having already been trained in both nursing and social work. Her objective was to become qualified as a medical practitioner so that she could more effectively work to improve the care of patients dying with cancer. Her efforts eventually bore fruit, and her goals were realized with the 1967 opening in London of St. Christopher's Hospice, the first of the modern hospices in the world.

Much has happened since the landmark Marie Curie Foundation study in 1951 and the opening of St. Christopher's in 1967. Today in the United States, there are more than 1,400 hospice programs and many additional programs that adhere to the basic principles of hospice care.[2] There are more than 64 hospice programs in Canada and an additional large number being considered or actually being organized.[3]

1. Marie Curie Memorial Foundation. A national survey concerning patients with cancer nursed at home. Marie Curie Memorial Foundation, London, 1952 April.

2. Joint Commission on Accreditation of Hospitals. JCAH hospice provider profile. Mimeo, JCAH, Chicago, 1984 June 20.

3. Southall, H. A survey of palliative care programmes and services in Canada. Mimeo, Palliative Care Foundation, Toronto, 1982 Dec.

What was merely a concept 20 years ago is now a growing, thriving, impressive collection of programs, workers, and resources that stretches across the United States. In many ways, the hospice concept has captured the imagination and the idealism of all sectors of American life to a degree that is quite remarkable for a society as heterogeneous as ours. Everyone seems to agree that the principles of hospice care for the dying are good and need to be implemented as widely as possible.

But how best to implement these principles? How many hospice programs are needed, and what should they look like? How should they be financed, and what sorts of standards of accountability should be imposed? How can the idealism and selfless dedication of the initial hospice developers be preserved in an era that has witnessed the development of more than a thousand new programs in a matter of several years?

Hospice work has moved into a new phase, a new generation — a phase in which these societal questions, these questions of public policy, require greater attention. The value of hospice programs is no longer debated; the question now is how this society can best respond to the challenge that is put forward by hospice programs for improved care for the dying.

This book has been developed to stimulate and to assist the important public policy debate that must surely take place if the principles of hospice care are to receive their appropriate attention and implementation. The book does not attempt to provide definitive answers for that debate, but rather tries to provide important questions that must be considered. The book is definitely pro hospice in the broadest sense but still attempts to maintain enough objectivity and thoughtful concern that it can question some of the basic assumptions and can challenge some of the basic tenets that have been central to hospice thinking since the beginning of modern hospice care.

The book has three sections, the first of which is devoted to certain background topics and is designed to ensure that all readers have the same basic knowledge of hospice programs in general. Chapter 1 surveys the origins and development of hospice programs in England, Canada, and the United States. Chapter 2 reviews the various forms and models of operation of hospice programs and considers the question of defining the term *hospice*. Chapter 3 summarizes available information about the current status of hospice programs in the United States.

The second section of the book looks at important issues in the consideration of future public policy for hospice programs. Chapter 4 asks, "Which dying patients should hospices serve?" Chapter 5, by Blum and Robbins, reviews questions of licensure for hospice programs. Chapter 6, by Tehan, is linked to the previous chapter on licensure and reviews questions of accreditation and standard-setting for hospice programs. Chapter 7, by Wales, examines the issue of evaluating hospice programs and provides some important considerations for future evaluation efforts.

Chapter 8, by Cummings, looks at financing of hospice programs, both what exists now and what will probably develop in the future. Chapter 9 examines issues of planning as they relate to hospice programs, both those issues related to the planning of individual hospice programs and also those issues that are important in areawide planning for health programs in general. In chapter 10, Lynn and Osterweis comment on important ethical issues related to hospice programs, and in chapter 11, English and Wilson discuss administrative and management questions of hospices.

Part 3 attempts to bring certain of the important public policy questions together in summary form. In chapter 12, Aiken and Marx provide an excellent overview of the important public policy issues about hospice programs and review some of the hard questions that hospice proponents must ask themselves in the near future, if they are to deal with that future successfully.

After the important aerial Battle of Britain in the second world war in which the embattled Royal Air Force turned back the threatening waves of German bombers, Winston Churchill was asked whether the British victory meant the end of the war. "No," he said, "it doesn't mean the end of the war; it is not even the beginning of the end of the war. However," he added reflectively, "it does mean the end of the beginning."

That is exactly where hospice programs in the United States now stand—at the end of their beginning phase. Now they are moving into a new, developmental phase that will present new challenges and call for new skills and leadership. How this new phase is handled may well decide the fate of hospice programs in this country for many years to come. It is hoped that this book will help the transition into that developmental phase so that it may be as smooth and as constructive as possible.

Paul R. Torrens

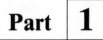

History and Background of Hospice Programs

Chapter 1

Development of Special Care Programs for the Dying: A Brief History

Paul R. Torrens, M.D., M.P.H.

The year was 1967, and in London and Chicago two remarkable women physicians were entering critical phases of their life's work, work that would revolutionize the care of the dying throughout the world. It would also lead to a massive reexamination of the purposes and practices of medical care.

Elisabeth Kübler-Ross

In Chicago, Elisabeth Kübler-Ross, M.D., a Swiss-born psychiatrist at the University of Chicago Hospital, was finishing nearly two years of conversations with dying patients and their families, during which time she had carefully and sympathetically tried to learn more about their plight. Working as a psychiatric liaison with medical and nursing staffs who were caring for the dying patients, she had come to understand a great deal about the psychological process of dying. She had also come to appreciate how little had actually been known about the thoughts and feelings of people facing death. As a result of her careful observations, she had documented the actual diminution of contacts between doctors and nurses and their patients once a terminal diagnosis was made, and she had gradually realized with horror that just at the time dying patients needed more attention and support, they actually seemed to receive less.

Her work had not been easy, however. Indeed, her own experiences in trying to get her research started told volumes about the American view of death in the mid-1960s. Writing later, she told how her work in Chicago began:

In the fall of 1965, four theology students of the Chicago Theological Seminary approached me for assistance in a research project they had chosen. Their class was to write a paper on "crisis in human life" and the four students considered death as the biggest crisis people had to face.

Finding patients for her students to interview, however, was quite another matter.

I set out to ask physicians of different services and wards for permission to interview terminally ill patients of theirs. The reactions were varied, from stunned looks of disbelief to rather abrupt changes of the topic of conversation....Some doctors "protected" their patients by saying that they were too sick, too tired or weak, or not the talking kind; others bluntly refused to take part in such a project.

It suddenly seemed that there were no dying patients in this huge hospital. My phone calls and personal visits to the wards were in vain. Some physicians said they did not wish to expose their patients to such questioning as it might tire them too much. A nurse angrily asked in utter disbelief if I enjoyed telling a 24-year-old man that he had only a couple of weeks to live.[1]

Kübler-Ross persisted, however, and gradually began to interview patients, their families, and the doctors and nurses working with them. Contrary to what she had been told in her initial search for patients to interview, she found these dying patients quite willing to talk about their plight and, indeed, quite eager to be heard. They provided her and her first four students (soon to be followed by many others) with a great volume of information about dying. They also pointed out to her and the students how inadequately the present methods of care were meeting their most critical personal needs.

In 1967, Kübler-Ross began to write down her findings, and in 1969 her book, *On Death and Dying,* landed with stunning effect on an unsuspecting and unprepared public. For one thing, it highlighted how little had previously been known about the process of dying, not only from the point of view of the patients but also, surprisingly enough, from the point of view of those who must care for them.

The book also showed that it was entirely possible to talk with the dying, to explore with them their most personal fears and feelings, and to conduct organized, disciplined research on dying just as one might carry out similar research on any other aspect of life. In addition, it pointed out the many therapeutic effects of letting dying patients talk about their situation, and it presented a number of important techniques by which doctors and nurses could help this process take place.

Perhaps just as important, Kübler-Ross's book presented a theoretical framework describing the psychological stages of dying, a model that allowed for a much closer and more exact understanding of patients and their needs. She suggested that dying patients passed through several transitions as they approached death, from denial and isolation ("No, not me; it can't be true"), to anger ("Why me?"), to bargaining ("I need more time!"), then to depression ("It's no use"), and finally to acceptance ("It won't be long now"). Although later work would challenge some aspects of this framework, for the moment it gave interested researchers and therapists an important beginning in their attempts to understand the dying patient better.

Throughout, *On Death and Dying* presented its readers with a warm and compellingly hopeful picture of a thoughtful physican working with dying patients to provide them with some personal peace before their end. Readers were attracted not just to the theoretical model of the psychology of the dying; they were also sympathetically drawn to the plight of dying patients and their families and were humanely stimulated to become interested in dying patients themselves. For many young physicians and nurses, reading *On Death and Dying* was an important milestone in their personal development, moving them along to a much better understanding of the humane purposes of their professions.

In addition, because of the widespread success of the book in both professional and lay circles, *On Death and Dying* shattered once and for all the taboo of not speaking openly and publicly about dying. It enabled interested laymen as well as professionals of all sorts to move past barriers of silence that had previously prevented much discussion or exchange of ideas. The intellectual integrity of the work encouraged thinkers and researchers to turn their attention toward the process of dying as a legitimate area of activity, while its warmly compassionate tone encouraged doctors, nurses, social workers, clergy, and others to look for better ways to serve patients. The wall of silence about death was broken down for good.

Cicely Saunders

Also in 1967, in London, an equally remarkable physician, Cicely Saunders, M.D., watched with pride as the object of her life's work, St. Christopher's Hospice, opened its doors. For many years she had worked for this moment, hoping to create a model program of care for the dying in which patients could find relief from their pain and professionals could find guidance in their work.

Originally trained as a nurse at the Nightingale School of St. Thomas's Hospital in London, she then took a degree in philosophy, politics, and economics at Oxford and the diploma in public administration. She did her practical training as a hospital almoner (social worker) and was then appointed assistant almoner at St. Thomas's in 1947. From 1948, she had the opportunity of regularly visiting St. Luke's Hospital in Bayswater, a hospital established in 1893 to care for those dying of cancer and tuberculosis.[2] The attitude of the staff, the standard of nursing, and control of pain were impressively better than anything she had seen in teaching and general hospitals, and the experience eventually led her to obtain medical training. She entered St. Thomas's Hospital Medical School in 1951 and qualified as a physician in 1957. After several years of fellowship in the Department of Pharmacology at St. Mary's Hospital Medical School, carrying out research into analgesics and other drugs used in the treatment of patients with terminal illness, she started to work at St. Joseph's Hospice in Hackney, a working-class section of London.

Founded in 1908 by the Irish Sisters of Charity, St. Joseph's had been providing traditional programs of nursing care for terminally ill patients for a long time. Now, under the inspiration of Saunders, new ideas of care began to emerge. Working intuitively, Saunders began to learn that control of pain was central to the care of the dying; without it, little else could be accomplished with the patient's other problems. She also learned how little was really known about the control of dying patients' pain and so began to experiment with new approaches toward relieving that pain. Saunders used higher doses of pain medications than had previously been thought possible and also provided this medication on a continuous basis in advance of pain and in anticipation of it rather than after it had already occurred, as had traditionally been the case. In this way, she began to understand better how to care for dying patients.

In adopting this approach to pain control, Saunders was building on some observations she had made 10 years earlier.

> (In 1948) I went as a volunteer SRN (state registered nurse) to St. Luke's Hospital in Bayswater. This was the first time I encountered the principle of overcoming constant pain with an equally constant control, by giving drugs regularly. They were used to prevent pain from occurring instead of to relieve it once it was present. (The hospital had in fact been using pain medication in this fashion since 1935.) I was immediately struck by the effectiveness of this method and the contrasts with my experience in general hospitals.[3]

The results were impressive. Dying patients at St. Joseph's became virtually pain-free, and Saunders was able to begin to work with their other emotional and personal problems. As Kübler-Ross would learn several years later in Chicago, Saunders learned that dying patients were quite capable of talking about their condition and indeed that they benefited considerably from the improved communication with their families and the staff taking care of them.

Whereas Kübler-Ross used her experience to develop a framework describing the transitional stages of dying, Saunders used hers to formulate a practical philosophy of caring for patients; she began to develop the basic elements that should comprise a model program for care of the dying. They included:

1. Management of the patient's care by a skilled, interdisciplinary team whose members communicate regularly with one another
2. Effective control of the common symptoms of terminal disease, especially pain in all its aspects
3. Recognition of the patient and the family as a single unit of care
4. An active home-care program
5. An active program of bereavement follow-up for the family following the death of the patient

Like Kübler-Ross, Saunders began in the 1960s to write about her experiences, but she chose to express herself in a string of insightful articles in medical and nursing journals rather than in a single book.[4-21] Speaking forcefully yet gently, she began to capture the interest of a small group of physicians and nurses throughout England and to build a personal network of colleagues and friends that would one day extend all over the world.

In 1967, Doctor Saunders was able to raise enough money from donations and other private sources to design and build a model hospice, St. Christopher's, in Sydenham on the outskirts of London. Set in a quiet residential neighborhood and designed specifically in all its aspects for the care of the dying, St. Christopher's became the embodiment of all of Saunders's personal and professional philosophies. Operating as a private charity, it contracted with the regional health authority of the National Health Service for the majority of its beds and thereby achieved a unique blend of the private institution's freedom to innovate and experiment and the government system's stability of financial support.

St. Christopher's was more than the site of remarkably effective programs of care for the dying; it also became a vigorous center for the training and education of health professionals from all over the world. Drawn by early reports of the work being conducted there, visitors came to St. Christopher's to witness what was being done and to report back to their friends and colleagues at home. In the United States, several of these visitors published their impressions of St. Christopher's in major professional journals, providing those who had read Kübler-Ross's book of 1969 with evidence that a better program of care for the dying was now available.

One of these visitors to St. Christopher's, Leonard Liegner, summarized in a report both the wonderment that such a program could exist and the desire that similar programs be developed in the United States.

Although I arrived with an initial resistance to continual contact with the dying patient, the actual experience was quite different from what I had expected. Instead of a terminal care or "death house" environment with cachectic, narcotized, bedridden, depressed patients, I found an active community of patients, staff, families, and children of staff and patients.

He went on to report:

The actual event of death is managed with dignity. The dying patient is not isolated behind curtains. All patients in the ward area are aware of what is transpiring. The lack of suffering, in fact the absolute absence of patient distress, is the unique factor permitting the staff and other patients to overcome their fear of death. This applies equally to families and children who, on visits the next day, note the passing of a previous patient whom they had befriended....The patient does not die alone and abandoned.

Finally, he summarized:

St. Christopher's Hospice teaches us that total care does not end when acute and chronic care are completed. The physician's "contract" with the patient extends to the management of his dying and his death and extends even beyond, to his surviving family. The hospice teaches a new attitude toward dying and death, with the realization and the conscious acceptance of dying and death as part of being born and part of the struggles of life.[22]

Liegner's report was also important in that it was published in the *Journal of the American Medical Association* and received widespread distribution and attention in medical circles throughout the country.

In the same fashion, another visitor to St. Christopher's, Florence Wald, summarized her experience for readers of the *American Journal of Nursing*.[23] Because she was a former dean of the school of nursing at Yale University and a leader in nursing education in the United States, her remarks commanded vigorous interest and respect in nursing circles throughout the country. Also, as was the case with Liegner's article in the *Journal of the American Medical Association*, the publication of Wald's views in the *American Journal of Nursing* ensured a nationwide audience of top leaders in the nursing profession.

For her part, in the late 1960s and early 1970s, Saunders entered upon an exhausting schedule of speaking and teaching engagements that took her across the Atlantic many times. In each of these important appearances, she encouraged her audiences not only to become more interested in the care of the dying but also to push for the development of new programs, new hospices in their own communities.

By the early 1970s, a solid foundation had been laid by the work of Kübler-Ross and Saunders. A tentative model of the psychological stages of dying had been developed by Kübler-Ross, and the vigorous interest of both professional and lay publics had been widely developed by her powerful book *On Death and Dying.* The basic principles of actual care of the dying had been effectively worked out by Saunders, and a model program based on these principles had actually been put into effect at St. Christopher's in London. Widespread lecturing and writing by both women had begun to stimulate broad interest in hospice programs and care of the dying all across England and the United States, and individuals in widely distant cities began to dream of developing hospice programs of their own.

Early Hospices in England and North America

At the time of the opening of St. Christopher's Hospice in 1967, there were only a few hospices in England and, for the most part, these had existed since the turn of the century: St. Joseph's in Hackney, Hereford Lodge (the former St. Luke's Hospital in Bayswater), and the Hospital of God in Clapham. The opening of St. Christopher's, however, spurred the interest of many people and organizations throughout England, and soon a number of hospices began making their appearance: St. Luke's Nursing Home in Sheffield, the Macmillan Unit of Christchurch Hospital in Christchurch, the Michael Sobell House of the Churchill Hospital in Oxford, and the various homes and centers established by the Marie Curie Foundation. Almost without exception, all of these first hospices were primarily inpatient programs, and the home care services were seen mostly as an adjunct or support to them.

In the United States and Canada, however, the first few programs that began to develop in the early 1970s were significantly different in organizational design from St. Christopher's, although they all drew their inspiration from that program. This difference would eventually cause some confusion in design and purposes, but in the beginning it was not a problem.

In 1975, after almost two years of discussion and planning, a Palliative Care Service was opened at the Royal Victoria Hospital in Montreal. It was of note in that it was not a separate freestanding building but was instead an integral part of the parent hospital. Although this was not the first such program in Canada, a similar unit having been established a short time earlier at St. Boniface Hospital in Winnipeg, the Royal Victoria Hospital rapidly became a very prominent program, both because of the vigor of its leadership and because of its affiliation with the Royal Victoria Hospital and the McGill University Medical School.

Located on one floor of the main hospital building, the inpatient unit included all the same services found at St. Christopher's but provided them in the context of a large, acute care general teaching hospital. The Palliative Care Service was complete and self-contained, but it had to coexist with all the other service units of the hospital and had to draw its support and staff from the same central sources as the rest of the units.

Describing the Palliative Care Service, the first director of the unit, Balfour Mount, M.D., discussed the advantages of the unit's location within the larger general hospital structure:

> One implication of the institutional location of a Palliative Care Service is the inherent accountability and peer review that such a setting provides. In addition, there are readily available consultants as well as diagnostic and therapeutic resources not found in freestanding hospices. A decompression laminectomy becomes an immediately available option for the acutely paretic patient; focal irradiation involves a stretcher ride down the hall rather than a trip by ambulance across town. The dermatologist may be asked to drop in during his regular hospital rounds to see the patient with a troublesome rash....
>
> It is not just the PCS that benefits from the service being within the institution. Experience suggests that the benefits go both ways. The presence of the PCS has led to an increased emphasis on whole-person medical care throughout the institution, in the opinion of independent evaluators within the Royal Victoria Hospital. Furthermore, since the transition from active anticancer treatment to palliative care is often unclear, difficult, or delayed, the presence of the PCS team within the institution is particularly useful since it facilitates their early involvement and lessens the trauma attached to this shift in therapeutic goals. When the decision is made that further treatment aimed at cure or prolonged life is inappropriate, it is frequently reassuring to the patient to know that the hospital has specialized facilities providing skill in symptom control and other aspects of his present needs and that he is not going to be discharged and "written off" by those previously involved in care, but transferred to a ward within the hospital where his own doctor can still visit regularly.[24]

At the same time as this program was developing in Montreal, the Hospice of Connecticut was starting to deliver care to dying patients in the New Haven area. The original plans were to construct a freestanding, purpose-built hospice much like St. Christopher's, but difficulties and delays in financing forced the hospice to begin as a home care, community service program. Much of the initial inspiration for the New Haven hospice came from Saunders herself, who took an active personal interest in its development.

Our (St. Christopher's) important links with the United States began in 1963, with an invitation to me from the Yale School of Medicine, through an English surgeon, Bernard Lytton, who had carried out a research project at St. Joseph's. Here I met Florence Wald, then dean of the graduate school of nursing at Yale who, when I was there again in 1966 as a visiting lecturer, invited Elisabeth Kübler-Ross, Colin Murray Parkes, and myself to meet in a workshop attended by others already involved in this field.[25]

Over the years, Saunders maintained a close interest in the developments in New Haven and eventually encouraged an English physician who had spent time in training at St. Christopher's, Sylvia Lack, M.D., to take on the responsibilities as medical director at the New Haven hospice after it opened in 1974.

In the beginning, the New Haven hospice operated no inpatient facility of its own but instead provided its program of care to patients in their own home or in the various acute care general hospitals of the community. After six years of operation, it finally was able to construct and open its own inpatient unit in 1980, but its early years as a home care program left an indelible impression on the purposes and practices of the hospice staff and administrators. It also provided the country with a new and different model of care for the dying, care that focused primarily on patients at home.

The early uncertainties about whether a home care hospice program would be successful in the United States were well articulated by Lack:

There was concern at the outset that palliative home care would be unacceptable in this country. I was frequently told that "Americans are hospital-oriented; when Americans are sick they want to be in a hospital." "Nobody dies at home in this country. The society is not set up for it."

Despite all these gloomy prophecies, hospice has demonstrated that home care is very much desired by a proportion of the population. Families are prepared to accept great hardship to keep a loved one home, and at the appropriate time, intensive personal care or palliative care at home is welcomed.[26]

About the same time in 1976 in Marin County, just north of San Francisco, a somewhat different variant of the home care model was being developed, incorporating unique features not present in any of the other programs previously developed, either in England, in Montreal, or in New Haven. First, the Hospice of Marin was largely sponsored and supported by enthusiastic lay workers (that is, nonmedical and nonnursing) who voluntarily donated their time and efforts to provide services to patients. In addition to the basically lay volunteer sponsorship of the program, the Hospice of Marin was also unique in that it had absolutely no intention of ever developing an inpatient facility of its own, either freestanding or as a part of a larger hospital. It was meant to be a volunteer supportive effort to caregivers already existing in the community and to their patients; it was not meant as an effort to supplant previous programs of care with an entirely new one.

The first medical director of the Hospice of Marin, William Lammers, M.D., gave some idea of challenges encountered by these early hospice program developers:

> At the beginning we learned that all of our previous professional education and experience was not sufficient to guarantee good hospice care for the dying. We had to learn new methods of controlling pain and symptoms in terminal illness. We had to come to better understandings of social, psychological, and spiritual aspects of death as they affected the dying person and the immediate family. We had to learn to communicate more openly with each other and with the dying, their families, and the professional community.

Indeed, the involvement of the family in the program of care was a major factor in the organization of the program in Marin, as Lammers made clear:

> We tried to involve families in providing care, and now feel that the time we spent in providing instruction, supervision, and round-the-clock support to families resulted in patients receiving excellent care in comfortable surroundings. We were, at the time, amazed at the ability of families and friends to learn to give careful attention to skin care, bathing, oral hygiene, record keeping, and general "comfort care." This participation showed us that the bereaved are able to show and give love and to feel after the death that they were able to contribute something special during the last days of their loved one.[27]

Once the Hospice of Marin was under way and largely because of its willingness to teach and educate others, a number of community-based, home care hospice programs began to develop around the country. In May 1977 the Hospice of Marin joined with the Hospice of New Haven and the Palliative Care Service of the Royal Victoria Hospital in sponsoring a "How-To of Hospice Care" conference in California, and representatives from 17 states attended.[28]

Although many of these community-based programs grew up without any preexisting organization sponsoring them, a number started within local visiting nurse services or home health agencies. In these latter hospices, there was usually some sort of organization already in existence, delivering nursing care and other supportive services to patients at home. Some of these organizations simply reorganized their packages of services, employed new personnel who were particularly interested in the care of the dying, and added certain new services (such as bereavement support and counseling). The advantages of having the previous organizational base from which to develop was highlighted by the remarks of Claire Tehan, who assisted in the development of one of the early programs of this type in the Hospital Home Health Care Agency of California.

A significant benefit of developing a hospice program within an existing home health care agency was the opportunity to share services and expertise of a variety of individuals. The hospice program has the opportunity to maximize its potential because of the resources available within the agency. When a hospice program functions within an existing agency, basic operational services (that is, switchboard, answering service, billing, typing, photocopying) can be shared.

A small hospice team can be augmented by other health care professionals working in the home care agency. Consultants are often a luxury that a hospice program cannot afford; in a home health agency, however, these individuals are often available for consultation and advice. An enterostomal therapist may be utilized as a consultant when a patient was having unusual difficulty with a colostomy. A pediatric nurse may be asked to visit a dying child and advise on a problem beyond the competence of the hospice team.

Likewise, a hospice staff person may offer consultation in pain control to a cancer patient who was receiving care in the regular home health program, since many of the techniques developed by the hospice team may be applicable to general medical-surgical patients. This also gives the hospice personnel a good opportunity to educate other health care professionals.

Tehan went on to point out:

There are often more patients who need hospice care than can be admitted to the program. A significant advantage to operating a hospice program within a home health agency was that those patients waiting to be admitted to the hospice program may still receive home care services from the regular medical-surgical program.

Likewise, there are always a number of patients whose condition stabilizes and who may not require the intensive services available to them through the hospice program. These patients can be transferred to the medical-surgical team for care until their condition deteriorates to the point at which hospice intervention was again appropriate.[29]

In 1977, the first freestanding inpatient hospice unit in the country was opened at the Hillhaven Hospice in Tucson, Arizona. Established by a foundation connected with a national proprietary nursing home organization and located in a former nursing home facility, it attempted to transplant the atmosphere and the organization of the London-based St. Christopher's to the southwestern desert climate of Arizona. There were difficulties in doing this, but a vigorous program was established and many new lessons were learned.[30]

Also in 1977, a final hospice model was developed at St. Luke's Hospital in New York City, a model that was different again from all the preceding ones. Interestingly enough, it was a model that would be transplanted back to England in 1978 to St. Thomas's Hospital in London.

In this type of hospice program, the "symptom control team" was the heart of the program, a team composed of skilled health care professionals who could be made available to all of the medical and nursing staff throughout the hospital for consultation and assistance with the problems of their patients. There was no special facility or location that clustered dying patients together, nor were there any specific personnel who would take on the total care of the dying patients on a full-time basis as in other hospice programs. Instead, the care of the dying patients was left in the hands of the regular hospital personnel; the symptom control team served to provide them with expert advice, assistance, and linkage with specialized sources of care outside the hospital.

In the minds of the developers of this variant of hospice care, the symptom control team provided a model that could be readily adapted in acute care general hospitals across the country at relatively low cost. In their eyes, if the care of the dying was to improve broadly across the country, a model program had to be developed that could be easily and readily inserted into the standard operations of the typical hospital and that could support the ordinary programs of care, not supplant them. As described by one of the early supporters of this variant of hospice:

> Hospice care should be part of the mainstream of American medicine and its institutions. Development of separate facilities for hospice care could be more costly and might result in the public perceiving hospices as another form of nursing home. Furthermore, hospital care should be influenced by the principles of hospice care; that is, caring and curing should be related....A hospice team or

consultant in every teaching hospital would enable today's students and tomorrow's health care providers to observe hospice care as an integral part of treatment in the acute care setting.[31]

By the end of 1977, six different models of hospice programs had been started in the United States and Canada, and much interest had been generated. Then, as the information about these initial programs here and in England began to spread, hospice programs began to appear at an astonishing rate.

Growth in Hospice Programs

The growth in numbers of hospice programs in England and in North America from 1977 onward has been impressive. Saunders began her work at St. Joseph's in Hackney in the late 1950s, and no major new project was developed in the care of the dying until she opened St. Christopher's Hospice in 1967. One by one, new projects were conceived and new programs opened all over the United Kingdom until, by the end of 1975, no fewer than 30 individual hospices were in operation.[32] A 1980 survey of hospice programs in Great Britain revealed a total of 70 separate units providing care to the dying, 58 of which were primarily inpatient units, 10 of which were primarily home care programs, and two of which were symptom control teams independent of an inpatient unit.[33-36]

In the United States, the growth has been even more explosive, particularly since 1977. Prior to that time, as had been the case in England before the opening of St. Christopher's, there had been only a very few units providing care for the dying, and these had been in existence for some years. The House of Calvary in the Bronx, the former Hospital of the Holy Ghost in Boston, and the various homes of the Hawthorne Dominican Sisters throughout New England had been providing sympathetic nursing care to dying patients for years but had received little attention. With the opening of the Hospice of Connecticut in New Haven in 1974, the Palliative Care Service at the Royal Victoria Hospital in Montreal in 1975, the Hospice of Marin in 1976, and the Hillhaven Hospice in 1977, a great upsurge of interest in the care of the dying and a vigorous burst of organizing activity occurred.

California provides a classic example of this explosive hospice development. In 1976, the Hospice of Marin opened and was followed quickly in the same year by several others. By 1977, there were eight hospices in some form of operation in California, and by 1978, a total of 16 were in existence.[37] When the scene was surveyed in early 1981, more than 67 separate units could be identified that were providing some form of care to the dying or planning to do so soon.[38] When the state was surveyed again in early 1984, a total of 166 operating hospices were found in California,[39] with 58 hospice programs in Southern California alone.[40]

Another example could be drawn from the experience of the Veterans Administration with regard to hospice programs and other programs for the terminally ill. Prior to 1978, the VA did not have a hospice program in any of its 170 hospitals, but in that year it authorized the first such program at the Wadsworth VA Hospital in Los Angeles. Four years later, in mid-1982, a survey showed that there were then 11 hospice or hospice-like programs in operation in the VA with another five proposed to begin within the next 12 months after the survey.[41]

This same pattern held true for the entire United States, although the figures are less clear because of difficulty in identifying and tabulating new programs. For example, the National Hospice Organization (NHO) was first brought together in 1973 with a handful of programs from around the country. By 1978, there were 63 hospice provider members, that is, programs actually giving hospice care or planning to do so within two years; by 1980 this number had risen to 135, and by 1982, there were 355 hospice programs in the NHO provider membership category.[42, 43]

In a survey carried out for the Joint Commission on Accreditation of Hospitals (JCAH) in early 1981, over 800 hospice programs were identified in various stages of development.[44] Of these, 440 individual hospices responded to a survey questionnaire, providing important information about themselves and their activities. Fifty-one percent of these 440 hospices stated that they had become operational only after January 1980. In a similar survey covering the states of Washington, Idaho, Oregon, and Montana in the United States and the province of British Columbia in Canada, researchers at the University of Washington found 32 operating hospices in January 1981 in the states and province covered, and another 10 that planned to open within the following year; the mean length of time that the 32 operational hospices had been in existence was 18 months.[45] When JCAH resurveyed the situation in early 1984, the number of hospices in the United States had gone from 800 to 1,429, and the number of hospices in Washington, Idaho, Oregon, and Montana had gone from 32 (including British Columbia) in 1981 to 83 (not including British Columbia) in 1984.[46]

The pattern of hospice development in Canada has been similar to that in the United States, at least in pace and size if not in the type of hospice programs developed. Following the opening of the first two units in Canada in 1975 at St. Boniface Hospital in Winnipeg and at the Royal Victoria Hospital in Montreal, a lot of interest in hospice care was generated throughout Canada. Most of this interest in Canada centered on hospitals, in contrast to the United States, where most of the initiative for new programs came from groups outside hospitals. As a result, the development of actual programs was initially slower in Canada than in the United States because there were more organizational constraints to be overcome.

By the late 1970s and early 1980s, however, these constraints were clearly no longer holding back the tide, and a significant number of hospice programs were in existence, with more being proposed. A survey conducted for the Palliative Care Foundation in Canada in 1982 disclosed that there were 64 hospice programs already operating and a further 18 to be implemented within 12 months from the time of the survey. An additional eight hospitals indicated a definite intention to implement a service in the near future and were working on the organizational details at the time of the survey.[47]

It is impossible to determine the exact number of hospice programs in the United States and Canada, as there is no required licensure or accreditation process for hospices that covers the entire country, nor is there any complete central registry for such programs. The JCAH survey probably represents the best estimate of hospice activity in the country, because it actively attempted to search out and identify all operational or prospective hospice programs in the country, but even this survey should be considered tentative at best.

The situation is even further complicated by the fact that there are additional patient care programs that provide many hospice-like services but that do not call themselves (or even consider themselves) hospices. These programs are generally component parts of comprehensive cancer centers and provide some or all of the services usually found in hospices. Whether these programs should be included in the hospice statistics and whether the definition of hospice should be broadened to include them are important questions for anyone attempting to measure the extent of the field at this time.

Societal Controls and Support in the United States

After 1980, the most important developments in the hospice movement in the United States were no longer just the growth in the number of hospice programs (although that growth continued unabated) or the developments in new forms of program. The important new developments in the hospice movement after 1980 were the beginning imposition of societal controls on hospice programs, on the one hand, and the initiation of societal support, on the other. The first development involved accreditation according to a preset collection of standards; the second involved the expansion of current federal health insurance (primarily Medicare) to cover hospice benefits.

For a number of years, hospice workers and the National Hospice Organization have been concerned about the standards of care to which any acceptable hospice should adhere. In 1979, a beginning set of standards for hospice programs was developed by NHO, and, as experience in the area grew, these standards were amended by NHO in 1981.[48, 49]

In mid-1981, the question of accreditation became a more important issue for hospice programs. Who would eventually decide what an acceptable hospice program is and what set of standards should be used? One set of regional efforts began in California under the auspices of the California Medical Association,[50] but a more national effort was developed by the Joint Commission on Accreditation of Hospitals with the support of a grant from the Kellogg Foundation. The JCAH effort included a national survey of hospice programs,[51] and, more important, included the development of a beginning process for evaluating and reviewing hospice programs against a predetermined set of standards.[52] These standards and the process of evaluating hospice programs according to these standards underwent extensive national testing and considerable effort and input from the hospice programs themselves. This resulted in a methodology for evaluating hospice programs that was approved by JCAH in 1983 and offered to hospices interested in seeking formal accreditation.[53]

At the same time as the development of accreditation processes (and indeed, probably giving rise to the urgency in developing those processes), coverage for hospice programs by various insurance mechanisms has grown. This has certainly been the most important development in hospice care since the initial creation of the first units in the mid-1970s, with the potential power to shape the hospice movement in the United States for many years to come.

In the early years of hospice program development in the United States, there was very little in the way of insurance or third-party payment to hospice programs for the care they were giving patients. Hospice programs were very largely viewed as extra care that was provided to patients as a community service by programs that were largely unaccredited, not specifically licensed, and generally not part of the recognized (and insurable) health care system.

As the years went by, small changes in this situation began to take place on both sides of the reimbursement fence. Individual hospice programs began to learn what they legitimately could bill insurance companies for, and they began to do so. Hospitals or home health agencies, for example, began to realize that although they might not be able to bill for a particular hospice service as "hospice," they could bill for that same service as part of the array of services they offered to all patients. Individual insurers, for their part, began to include hospice benefits in their plans or began to expand the definition and the application of some of their existing coverages that bordered on the area served by hospices. A number of large corporations (such as Westinghouse, Radio Corporation of America, and General Electric) began to add hospice benefits to their insurance packages, and a number of the insurance carriers (Blue Cross, most notably) began to offer broader hospice coverage as well.

Certainly the most significant development in this area was the introduction of a bill in Congress in the summer of 1982 that specifically added hospice coverage to those services already provided under the federal Medicare program. Although the prospects of any new additions to the federal Medicare program at this time of economic constraints seemed to be very unlikely, the legislation introduced by Representative Leon Panetta (D-CA) in the House of Representatives and by Senator Robert Dole (R-KS) in the Senate passed with overwhelming support, not only ensuring inclusion for hospice care in the Medicare program but also visibly signalling the strong support by Congress for this type of health care.[54] Although the implementation of this benefit has been complex, as described in more detail in chapter 8, hospice care has entered into the mainstream of health care financing, if not provision, in the United States.

Rapid Spread of Hospice Concept

Why has there been this great explosion of interest in hospice programs? What caused this rapid spread of the idea and the widespread development of these new programs?

There were several obvious factors that helped spur this development. First, a number of physicians from England who are very effective speakers (Cicely Saunders, Thomas West, and Colin Murray Parkes from St. Christopher's and Richard Lamerton from St. Joseph's, among others) repeatedly made major speaking tours through the United States, attracting large numbers of enthusiastic listeners. They were able to imbue their listeners with their own sense of special purpose and idealism, which the listeners then passed along to others.

In particular, Saunders devoted a great deal of time and energy to identifying potential sources of leadership for the hospice movement and potential sites for future hospices. She actively encouraged those early leaders to make their hopes for hospice a reality and provided them with expert advice and assistance whenever possible. The amount of time and energy she devoted to this early nurturing effort and her willingness to expend herself in this role can well be seen from this excerpt from the St. Christopher's 1977-1978 Annual Report:

> This year (1977), we have had several contacts with the National Cancer Institute, USA. I paid a brief visit to discuss the principles of hospice care, today's standards and the challenge of evaluating their interpretation in different settings. I left St. Christopher's at 10:00 a.m. on Monday and, flying by Concorde, was lecturing by 3:30 p.m. their time. After a working supper and a day's discussion on evaluation, I returned overnight in a 747 and was back in

the hospice by noon. After dealing with the post I staggered home, slept 15 hours straight off and by Thursday morning hardly felt I had been away.[55]

Also, large numbers of Americans were traveling to England, first to St. Christopher's and St. Joseph's, then later to other centers as they opened: St. Luke's in Sheffield, Michael Sobell House in Oxford, the Countess Mountbatten Home in Southampton, St. Columba's in Edinburgh. There, they were universally received with courtesy and enthusiasm for the hospice cause, enthusiasm that they brought back with them to the United States in their reports to colleagues and friends on their return. In 1977 alone, St. Christopher's had a total of 3,802 visitors for half-days or days, and 90 "resident" visitors-in-training for longer periods of time. During that year, 267 physicians paid day visits to St. Christopher's, as did 14 medical students.[56]

This was not to say that hospice leaders in the United States and Canada were not doing their part as well. Indeed, the early centers that were developing in Montreal, in New Haven, in Marin County, and in Tucson felt obligated to share their experiences with colleagues from across the country who wanted to see what they were doing. This often imposed a major obligation on these programs because just at the time that they were struggling to get organized to deliver services, they were receiving large numbers of requests for training and orientation from others.

In addition to these factors, there was also a mushrooming growth of the professional literature, as well as a great interest by the lay press and other media about this new area of concern. Balfour Mount, Ina Ajemian, and Ronald Melzack from the Royal Victoria Program produced many significant papers for the professional journals,[57-69] as did Sylvia Lack, Robert Buckingham, and Florence Wald in New Haven.[70-87] Sandol Stoddard's book *The Hospice Movement: A Better Way of Caring for the Dying*[88] and Sylvia Lack's and Robert Buckingham's book *First American Hospice*[89] were very well received and were soon followed by others by Rossman, Davidson, Cohen, DuBois, and Koff.[90-94]

A significant development in these early years was the formation in 1973 of an informal association, the National Hospice Organization, under the leadership of Dennis Rezendes from New Haven and Zachary Morfogen from the Riverside Hospice in Boonton, New Jersey. In 1977, the National Hospice Organization was formally incorporated, and in 1978 the first annual NHO meeting was held in Washington, DC, attended by 1,000 people. At that meeting, the Secretary of Health, Education, and Welfare, Joseph Califano, gave the keynote address and encouraged the active development of the hospice movement in the United States.[95]

In retrospect, it is difficult to determine whether the development of hospice programs stimulated the interest of the general public in death and dying, or whether the impetus came from the other direction (that is, increased public interest in death and dying made possible broad-scale support for, and interest in, hospice programs). Regardless of which came first, it is important to note that the two currents of interest — one (among the lay public) in the general aspects of death and dying and the other (among the health professionals) in the specific aspects of care for the dying — were taking place side by side, with each feeding and supporting the other in ways that had not been possible in previous years.

Government Support in the United States and Canada

At the same time, there has been considerable direct and indirect government support in both Canada and the United States. The first hospice program in the United States, in New Haven, Connecticut, received considerable financial support from the National Cancer Institute of the U.S. National Institutes of Health, as did three other hospice programs sponsored by the Kaiser-Permanente Health Plan in southern California, the Hillhaven Hospice in Tucson, Arizona, and the Riverside Hospice in Boonton, New Jersey.[96] In an early stage of hospice development in the United States, when education of the public and of policymakers was important, the U.S. General Accounting Office issued a background summary on hospice programs that was influential in gaining acceptance for hospice as a legitimate type of health care program.[97]

Also at an early stage of hospice development in the United States, both California and New York authorized special pilot projects to explore further the implications of hospice care for the people of those states.[98, 99] In 1980, the U.S. Health Care Financing Administration joined together with the Robert Wood Johnson Foundation and the John A. Hartford Foundation to sponsor a national study on hospice programs and their need for better financial support. In the summer of 1982, when Congressman Panetta and Senator Dole were introducing legislation in the Congress to broaden the Medicare insurance coverage to include hospice services, the Congressional Budget Office issued a report that suggested that coverage of hospice programs under Medicare could lead to considerable financial savings, if such coverage was properly designed and administered.[100] At the same time in Canada, the Policy, Planning, and Information Branch of the Department of National Health and Welfare was issuing a report that suggested that "if a national home care program for the terminally ill were coupled with the promotion of special palliative care units within hospitals to meet the needs of one-third of patients remaining in hospitals, the net cost savings could top $700 million per year."[101] This followed another publication by the Department of National Health and Welfare almost a year earlier in 1981, which set out guidelines

for the establishment of palliative care services in hospitals, thereby implying that it was encouraging the development of such services.[102] Clearly
the government role in support of the development of hospice programs,
even if primarily indirect, has been substantial, timely, and very important.

Additional Influences on Hospice Development

There are several points in this historical development that should be
emphasized, as they help explain why the present hospice programs exist
and operate in the form and manner they do.

First, it must be remembered that many of the initial hospice programs in the United States developed outside hospitals and, in some cases,
in spite of them. Hospitals in the United States were generally not interested
in the care of the dying and in some instances were actively hostile to the
idea of special care for the dying.

This lack of hospital interest in the special care of the dying forced
the early American hospice programs to look elsewhere for support and
encouragement. Early hospice workers felt that the success or failure of
their programs depended entirely upon the hospice workers themselves,
because they could not count on the support or assistance of hospitals.
The hospice workers were forced to develop a spirit of resolute independence that they might not have developed if they had been lulled by the
promise of protective support by a parent institution.

Also, because most of the early U.S. hospice programs developed
independently of hospitals, there was no traditional or conservative force
restraining their sense of innovation. There was usually no long-established
organization present to say, "In our experience, you really should not take
on that particular activity." Indeed, since most hospice programs saw their
whole existence as an innovation, a new direction, they almost felt obliged
to experiment with new approaches to patient care that might not have
been tolerated elsewhere.

In addition, because hospitals and much of the health care establishment were not interested in the early hospice programs, the leadership of
these programs often fell to interested lay and non-health-care personnel.
People without prior health care training or experience, who in a traditional hospital setting would not have been allowed to participate very
actively in the patient care process, were able to take the lead in the development of the new hospice programs. To this day, even though all good
hospice programs have physician and nurse participation, much of the
leadership and motivational force comes from nonprofessionals and from
the general public.

Unfortunately, this lack of hospital involvement has had some negative effects as well. It has fostered a somewhat antihospital and sometimes antidoctor attitude among hospice workers. Because of their

"refugee" status in general, many hospice workers have significant antipathy toward hospitals and sometimes toward doctors, a background that colors the hospice programs' attitudes toward the more established aspects of health care. It should not be too surprising that many hospice workers actively resist any discussion of integration of hospice programs into the traditional health care system of this country.

A further negative result of this isolation from hospitals involves the financial organization of today's hospice programs. Because the early hospice programs were not covered by health insurance and because they depended very heavily on volunteer workers and donated equipment, very little attention was really given to the financial affairs of hospices. Not much real planning effort was devoted to the financial futures of the programs, nor were adequate systems of accounting and financial management established.

As a result, as more and more hospice services begin to be covered by health insurance plans today and as more and more public and private organizations want to know the actual costs of providing hospice care, the programs themselves are frequently ill-equipped to furnish the necessary information. Hospice programs have made great strides in their patient care activities over the years, but they are still rather rudimentary "country store" operations as far as their finances are concerned. This might not have happened if hospitals, with their longer experience in health care financial management, had been more actively involved in the beginning.

A second major feature of the development of hospices has been the rapidity with which they have sprung up all over the country almost at the same time. In the mid-1970s, there were probably no more than a dozen hospice programs throughout the United States and Canada. By the late 1970s, there were possibly as many as 50 hospices, either actually delivering services or getting organized to do so. By the early 1980s, there were probably 500 operational programs in the United States and Canada, with several hundred more getting ready to deliver services; by 1984, the number was well over 1,400 such programs.

Because of the rapid development of these programs, there was no opportunity to collect and distribute information or to develop any accepted standards or operating norms. Interested parties had probably read about St. Christopher's and possibly one or two of the other early hospice programs in England, and they had probably heard one or two speakers describing their early efforts, but there simply was no long tradition of operating in a certain fashion or format. There were no widely accepted guidelines and no long record to which interested people could refer early in the development of these programs.

As a result, hospice programs plunged ahead in their development without any established pattern or guidelines of what the programs should really be, how they should be financed, or how they should fit into an already existing health care system. The enthusiastic supporters of these programs were so captured by the idea of hospice and so anxious to get them established and operating that they spent little time in any long-range planning or thought for the future. They merely worked hard, designed their programs, and brought them into existence as quickly as they could.

Because of this swift development, certain important questions that probably should have been raised *before* hospice programs became established simply were not asked: Is this program actually needed in this area? How many such programs do we need in this city, state, or country? How should these programs be financed over the long haul? How shall we go about licensing hospice programs to ensure that they meet some sort of standard? How do we go about telling a good program from one that is not so good? How do we develop support and linkages for these programs with hospitals, doctors, health insurance plans, and public health departments already in existence in the community?

This is not to say that hospice programs *should* have waited until all these questions were answered before they developed. Indeed, if they had waited for that type of traditional development, they most likely would never have developed with the vigor and unrestrained enthusiasm that has been characteristic of them up to this point.

Unfortunately, however, this country must now start to address some of these major policy questions concerning hospice programs, long after the programs themselves have come into existence and have established their pattern of operation. It will be much more difficult to view some of these important questions with any degree of objectivity, because there are now many vigorous and vocal adherents of hospice programs who have a strong vested interest in keeping their programs just the way they are.

Putting the genie back into the bottle after it has once emerged is very difficult, and attempting to develop clear and objective answers to the important public policy questions regarding hospices after so many of them have already come into existence will be equally difficult. However, it is in the genuine best interest of both the public that is served by these programs and the hospice programs themselves that these important policy questions be addressed directly and vigorously.

References

1. Kübler-Ross, E. *On Death and Dying.* New York: Macmillan Publishing Co., 1969.
2. Goldin, G. A protohospice at the turn of the century: St. Luke's House, London, from 1893 to 1921. *Journal of the History of Medicine and Allied Sciences.* 1981. 36:383-415.
3. Saunders, C. Control of pain in terminal cancer. *Nursing Times.* 1976 July 1.
4. Saunders, C. Management of patients in the terminal stage. In: Raven, R. W., editor. *Cancer,* vol. 6. London: William Heineman Medical Books, 1958.

5. Saunders, C. Care of the dying. *Nursing Times* reprint. London: Macmillan Publishing Co., 1960.

6. Saunders, C. Treatment of intractable pain in terminal cancer. *Proceedings of the Royal Society of Medicine.* 1963. 56:191-97.

7. Saunders, C. The symptomatic treatment of malignant disease. *Prescriber's Journal.* 1964. 4:68-70.

8. Saunders, C. The last stages of life. *American Journal of Nursing.* 1965. 65:432-35.

9. Saunders, C. The need for institutional care for the patient with advanced cancer. In: *Anniversary Volume, Madras Cancer Institute.* Madras, India: MCI, 1964.

10. Saunders, C. Telling patients. *District Nursing.* 1965. 8:149-50.

11. Saunders, C. Watch with me. *Nursing Times.* 1965. Nov. 26.

12. Saunders, C. The care of the dying. *Guy's Hospital Gazette.* 1966. 80:136-37.

13. Saunders, C. Death and responsibility: A medical director's view. *Psychiatric Opinion.* 1966. 3:28-34.

14. Saunders C. The management of terminal illness. *Hospital Medicine.* Part 1, 1966 Dec. 225-28. Part 2, 1967 Jan. 317-20. Part 3, 1967 Feb. 433-36.

15. Saunders, C. Terminal patient care. *Geriatrics.* 1966. 21:70-74.

16. Saunders, C. The care of the terminal stages of cancer. *Annals of the Royal College of Surgeons.* 1967. 41:162-64.

17. Saunders, C. The management of fatal illness in childhood. *Proceedings of the Royal Society of Medicine.* 1969. 62:549-54.

18. Saunders, C. The nursing of patients dying of cancer. *Nursing Times.* 1969. 55:1091-92.

19. Saunders, C. A therapeutic community: St. Christopher's hospice. In: Schoenberg, B., and others. *Psychosocial Aspects of Terminal Care.* New York: Columbia University Press, 1972.

20. Saunders, C. A death in the family: A professional view. *British Medical Journal.* 1973 Jan. 6. 30-31.

21. Saunders, C., and Winner, A. Research into terminal care of cancer patients. In: *Portfolio for Health: The Developing Program of the D.H.S. in Health Services Research. Problems and Progress in Medical Care,* vol. 8. Published for the Nuffield Provincial Hospitals Trust. London: Oxford University Press, 1973.

22. Liegner, L. St. Christopher's hospice, 1974. Care of the dying patient. *Journal of the American Medical Association.* 1975. 234:1047-48.

23. Craven, J., and Wald, F.S. Hospice care for dying patients. *American Journal of Nursing.* 1975. 75:1816-22.

24. Mount, B., and Ajemian, I. The palliative care service integration in a general hospital. In: Ajemian, I., and Mount, B., editors. *The Royal Victoria Hospital Manual on Palliative/Hospice Care.* New York: Arno Press, 1980.

25. Saunders, C. Annual report—St. Christopher's Hospice, Sydenham, England, 1977-1978.

26. Lack, S. New Haven (1974). Characteristics of a hospice program of care. *Death Education.* 1978. 2:41-52.

27. Lammers, W. Marin County (1976). Development of the hospice of Marin. *Death Education.* 1978. 2:53-62.

28. Lammers.

29. Tehan, C. Hospice in an existing home care agency. *Family and Community Health.* 1982. 5:11-20.

30. Hackley, J. Tucson (1977). Hillhaven Hospice. *Death Education.* 1978. 2:63-82.

31. Sweetser, C. Integrated care: The hospital-based hospice. *Quality Review Bulletin.* 1979. 5(5):18-22.

32. Hospices in the United Kingdom. *Nursing Times.* 1976 July 1.

33. Lunt, B. Terminal cancer care: Specialist services available in Great Britain in 1980. Survey report, Wessex Regional Cancer Organization and the University of Southampton, 1981 Mar.

34. Lunt, B. Terminal care services in Great Britain: The current picture and future developments. St. Christopher's Hospice, Sydenham, England, 1983.

35. Lunt, B., and Hillier, R. Terminal care: Present services and future priorities. *British Medical Journal.* 1981 Aug. 283:595-98.

36. Taylor, H. *The Hospice Movement in Britain: Its Role and Its Future.* London: Center for Policy on Aging, 1983.

37. Klutch, M. Hospices for terminally ill patients. *Western Journal of Medicine.* 1978. 129:82-84.

38. Falknor, H. P., and Kugler, D. JCAH hospice project, interim report: Phase I. Mimeo, Joint Commission on Accreditation of Hospitals, Chicago, 1981 July.

39. Joint Commission on Accreditation of Hospitals. JCAH hospice provider profile. Mimeo, JCAH, Chicago, 1984 June 20.

40. Hospice Organization of Southern California. Membership records, Los Angeles, 1984 Mar.

41. Chief Medical Director's Letter (IL 10-82-23). Department of Medicine and Surgery, Veterans Administration. Washington, DC, 1982 June 10.

42. National Hospice Organization. Annual report to the membership of the National Hospice Organization, 1980. McLean, VA, 1980.

43. National Hospice Organization. Annual report to the membership of the National Hospice Organization, 1982. Arlington, VA., 1982.

44. Falknor and Kugler.

45. Long-Term Care Gerontology Center. Survey results: The diversity and research interest of hospices in the northwest. Mimeo, University of Washington, 1981 Jan.

46. Joint Commission on Accreditation of Hospitals. JCAH hospice provider profile.

47. Southall, H. A survey of palliative care programmes and services in Canada. Mimeo, Palliative Care Foundation, Toronto, 1982 Dec.

48. National Hospice Organization. *Standards of a Hospice Program of Care,* 6th revision. McLean, VA: NHO, 1979.

49. National Hospice Organization. *Revised Principles and Standards of Hospice Care.* Arlington, VA: NHO, 1981.

50. Hospice accreditation criteria, preliminary working draft. Mimeo, Bay Area Hospice Association (San Francisco)-California Medical Association-Southern California Hospice Association, San Francisco, 1982 June 18.

51. Falknor and Kugler.

52. Joint Commission on Accreditation of Hospitals. Hospice project standards, preliminary working draft. Mimeo, JCAH, Chicago, 1982 Feb.

53. Joint Commission on Accreditation of Hospitals. *Hospice Standards Manual.* Chicago: JCAH, 1983.

54. H.R. 5180, 97th Congress of the United States (lst session). To amend Title XVIII of the Social Security Act to provide the coverage of hospice care under the Medicare Program. Panetta, L., Pepper, C., Waxman, H., Rangel, C., Gephardt, R., Conable, B., Gradison, W., and Madigan, E., 1981 Dec. 11.

55. Saunders. Annual report – St. Christopher's Hospice.

56. Saunders. Annual report – St. Christopher's Hospice.

57. Melzack, R. and others. The Brompton mixture effects on pain in cancer patients. *Canadian Medical Journal.* 1976. 115:125-29.

58. Mount, B., and others. Death and dying: Attitudes in a teaching hospital. *Urology.* 1974. 4:741.

59. Mount, B. Improving the Canadian way of dying. *Ontario Psychologist.* 1975. 7:19.

60. Melzack, R. The McGill pain questionnaire: Major properties and scoring methods. *Pain.* 1975. 1:277.

61. Mount, B. Palliative Care Service: October 1976 report. Royal Victoria Hospital-McGill University, Montreal, Canada, 1976.

62. Mount, B., Ajemian, I., and Scott, J. Use of the Brompton mixture in treating the chronic pain of malignant disease. *Canadian Medical Association Journal.* 1976. 115:122-24.

63. Mount, B. The problem of caring for the dying in a general hospital: The palliative care unit as a possible solution. *Canadian Medical Association Journal.* 1976. 115:119-21.

64. Mount, B., Melzack, R., and MacKinnon, K. J. The management of intractable pain in patients with advanced malignant disease. *Journal of Urology.* 1978. 120:720-25.

65. Munro, S., and Mount, B. Music therapy in palliative care. *Canadian Medical Association Journal.* 1978. 119:1029-34.

66. Wilson, D. C., Ajemian, I., and Mount, B. Montreal (1975). The Royal Victoria Hospital Palliative Care Service. *Death Education.* 1978. 2:3-19.

67. Ajemian, I. An oral morphine mixture for intractable pain. *Canadian Family Physician.* 1977. 23:1506-7.

68. Life and death in the palliative care unit: Montreal's Royal Victoria Hospital. *Dimensions in Health Service.* 1975. 52:22-25.

69. Mount, B. Palliative care of the terminally ill. *Annals of the Royal College of Physicians and Surgeons of Canada.* 1978. 76:201-6.

70. Lack, S., and Buckingham, R. *First American hospice: Three Years of Home Care.* New Haven, CT: Hospice Inc. 1978.

71. Lack, S. Death with dignity at home. *The Washington Post.* 1975 Nov. 16.

72. Dobihal, E. Talk or terminal care? *Connecticut Medicine.* 1974. 38:364-67.

73. Buckingham, R., Lack, S., and others. Living with the dying: Use of the technique of participant observation. *Canadian Medical Association Journal.* 1976. 115:1211-15.

74. Dobihal, E., Lack, S., and others. *Principles of Hospice Care.* New Haven, CT: Hospice, Inc. 1975.

75. Buckingham, R. Primary care of the terminally ill. *Geriatrics.* 1979. 34:73-75.

76. Dobihal, S. V. Hospice enables a patient to die at home. *American Journal of Nursing.* 1980. 80:1448-51.

77. Lack, S. Hospice—A concept of care in the final stage of life. *Connecticut Medicine.* 1979. 43:67-72.

78. Buckingham, R., and Foley, S. H. A guide to evaluation research in terminal care programs. *Death Education.* 1978. 2:41-52.

79. Lack, S. New Haven (1974). Characteristics of a hospice program of care. *Death Education.* 1978. 2:41-52.

80. Lack, S. I want to die while I'm still alive. *Death Education.* 1977. 1:165-76.

81. Buckingham, R. Hospice and health policy. *Health Policy Education.* 1980. 1:303-15.

82. Lack, S. Hospice helps patients 'live until they die.' *Hospital Administration Currents.* 1978. 22:27-30.

83. Foster, Z., Wald, F., and Wald, H. The hospice movement: A backward glance at its first two decades. *New Physician.* 1978. 27:21-24.

84. Craven, J., and Wald, F. Hospice care for dying patients. *American Journal of Nursing.* 1975. 75:1816-22.

85. Lack, S. Philosophy and organization of a hospice program. In: Garfield, C., editor. *Psychosocial Care of the Dying.* San Francisco: University of California Press, 1976.

86. Wald, F. Terminal care and nursing education. *American Journal of Nursing.* 1979. 79:1762-64.

87. Wald, F., Foster, Z., and Wald, H. The hospice movement as a health care reform. *Nursing Outlook.* 1980. 28:173-78.

88. Stoddard, S. *The Hospice Movement: A Better Way of Caring for the Dying.* New York: Stein and Day, 1978. London: Jonathan Cope, 1979.

89. Lack and Buckingham. *First American Hospice.*

90. Rossman, P. *Hospice: Creating New Models of Care for the Terminally Ill.* New York: Association Press, 1977.

91. Cohen, K. *Hospice: Prescription for Terminal Care.* Germantown, MD: Aspen Systems Corporation, 1979.

92. Davidson, G. W., editor. *The Hospice: Development and Administration.* Washington, DC: Hemisphere Publishing Corporation, 1978.

93. Koff, T. H. *Hospice: A Caring Community.* Cambridge, MA: Winthrop Publishing, Inc., 1980.

94. DuBois, P. M. *The Hospice Way of Death.* New York: Human Science Press, 1979.

95. Califano, J. Secretary Califano pledges support of hospice movement. *Aging.* 1978 Nov.-Dec.

96. A cost analysis of three programs: Hospice — Comprehensive cost analysis and executive summary. Kaiser-Permanente Medical Care Program, Los Angeles, 1981 July.

97. General Accounting Office. *Report to Congress: Hospice Care — A Growing Concept in the United States.* (HRD 79-50). Washington, DC: U.S. Government Printing Office, 1979.

98. Farley, H. Hospice: Its concept and legislative development. Report of the New York State Senate Committee on Aging, Albany, NY, 1982 Sept.

99. California Department of Health Services. Palliative care service pilot project. Report to the 1980 California legislature on the hospice project pursuant to Assembly Bill 1586, CH 1324, 1978, Sacramento, 1980.

100. Congressional Budget Office cost estimates. Washington, DC: Congressional Budget Office, 1982 June 28.

101. Department of National Health and Welfare. Policy, Planning, and Information Branch. *Palliative Care in Canada.* Ottawa, Canada: DNHW, 1982 Sept.

102. Department of National Health and Welfare. Health Services Directorate. Health Services and Promotion Branch. *Palliative Care Services in Hospitals: Guidelines for Establishing Standards for Special Services in Hospitals.* Ottawa, Canada: DNHW, 1981.

Chapter | **2**

More Than Semantics: What Is a Hospice?

Paul R. Torrens, M.D., M.P.H.

On all sides, one reads of new hospice programs being started, new legislation being drafted that will directly affect the future of the hospice movement, of new research being planned or actually conducted into the costs or effectiveness of hospice programs. The assumption could easily be made that the term *hospice* is being used to describe a single universe of institutions and programs that share a great similarity in their purpose, organization, and function.

This is misleading, for although hospice programs share a common purpose (that is, the improved care of the dying), they may differ widely from one another in the way they achieve that purpose. Indeed, at times the differences between individual hospice programs in the United States seems to be much more striking than their similarities.

Defining *hospice* therefore becomes more than a simple problem in semantics. Not all hospice programs are the same, and a clear understanding of their differences is important for the development of appropriate public policy regarding them in the future.

Hospital Models

The hospice model upon which most of the early programs were based, at least in their internal array of services, was St. Christopher's Hospice at Sydenham in London. Its originator, Cicely Saunders, M.D.,wanted to develop a facility that could be devoted completely and entirely to the care of the dying and also one that would be free of the usual pressures and problems of ordinary hospital life. For these reasons, she planned and built a new freestanding facility that was not connected in any way with a hospital or any other facility. She felt that the hospice idea was in some ways too fragile and uncertain a thing to withstand the uninformed criticism and scepticism that was sure to come, and that the infant idea might simply never get a fair chance to develop and flourish unless it had a place of its own. She had also seen the freedom that the older freestanding facilities at St. Joseph's in Hackney and St. Luke's in Bayswater had enjoyed because of their separate status, and she was determined to have this same freedom to innovate in her new hospice, St. Christopher's.[1]

As a result, the first modern hospice in England was a separate facility, one to which patients were transferred from other hospitals and health care programs in the area. When St. Christophers's was followed by the development of a second excellent freestanding facility, St. Luke's Nursing Home in Sheffield, under the inspiration and guidance of Professor Eric Wilkes, the image of the hospice as a separate entity was further reinforced. Because these two early hospices also became major teaching centers for hospice work and were visited by large numbers of the early leaders in hospice work around the world, it was only natural that the image of a hospice as a freestanding building would be widely promulgated.

It soon became evident in England, however, that the development of completely freestanding and separate facilities might not be feasible in any large numbers; it also became apparent that there were some considerable disadvantages to being cut off from the ordinary support services found in hospitals and to being so distant from the original source of patients. A freestanding hospice that operates at any distance from its hospital source of patients is frequently not able to intervene early in the process of identification and referral of suitable patients, with the result that the caring process of the hospice starts somewhat later in the course of an illness than it should. A freestanding hospice must also either develop its own competence in laboratory, x-ray, and other ancillary services or make some arrangements for obtaining them from other facilities whenever needed.

These realities influenced the development of the next few hospices in England in such a way that they were built as freestanding, self-contained units located on the grounds of general hospitals of one kind or another. The Michael Sobell House on the grounds of the Churchill Hospital at Oxford, the Countess Mountbatten Home on the grounds of the Moorgreen Hospital in Southampton, and the Christchurch Hospice on the grounds of the general hospital in Christchurch were all examples of this model, built with the help of large developmental grants from the National Society for Cancer Relief.

These hospices had the advantage of being separate, distinct entities within the hospital complex, remaining free to set their own patient care policies and procedures and yet being able to easily draw upon the resources of the hospital and its staff whenever necessary. The hospices were able to interact more easily with the hospital medical staff in identifying suitable patients and in facilitating their eventual referral to the hospice unit. In another area, these hospices were able to begin educating and proselytizing the hospital medical and nursing staffs in ways that a more distant freestanding hospice could not. Simply by being present within the hospital complex, the personnel in these hospices had more frequent access to people and patients than the original freestanding models.

Almost immediately, however, these second-wave hospice programs in England were faced with the same reality that had confronted their predecessors: once the initial development money for these model "Mac-Millan Units" from the National Society for Cancer Relief was exhausted, it was unlikely that the National Health Service would be able to construct a large number of such hospital-based freestanding units either. If more programs for the care of the dying were to be developed in England and in other countries, new organizational models would have to be considered that did not depend so heavily on the initial investment of large amounts of money for the construction or renovation of buildings.

At this point, two separate streams of hospice programs began to develop, one within hospitals and the other outside hospitals in the community at large. This dual stream of hospice programs and hospice philosophy continues and forms one of the major divisions in hospice policy and politics to this day.

On the hospital side, a group of creative workers at the Royal Victoria Hospital in Montreal, Canada, under the energetic leadership of Balfour Mount, M.D., were able to get a specific nursing unit of the hospital designated for the care of only terminally ill patients. Within this unit, the special staff members assembled for the project were able to offer their patients essentially the same type of care that was offered by the freestanding hospice programs in England but were able to do it directly within a general hospital. Several other hospitals in the United States and Canada developed this type of model, including the Kaiser-Permanente Hospice in the Kaiser Hospital in Hayward, California; the Parkwood Community Hospital in the San Fernando Valley in California; St. Boniface Hospital in Winnipeg, Canada; and the Palliative Care Unit in the Wadsworth Veterans Administration Hospital in Los Angeles, California.

In a number of hospitals, however, interested personnel were not able to develop even this type of program, and they felt quite frustrated in their attempts to improve the care of the dying within their hospitals. Many of these hospitals did not have a nursing unit available for conversion into a hospice program. Either all the hospital beds were full and it seemed impossible to reassign a significant number of them to the care of the dying, or the hospital administration was worried about the cost of operating such a specialized unit with its unknown chances for success.

Also in some of these hospitals, there was frequently significant resistance from medical staffs (and sometimes nursing staffs) who were reluctant to turn over the care of their patients to some new and entirely different team of doctors and nurses. They were hesitant about transferring their patients away to an untried and untested "death unit" and discouraged the development of such new units.

As a result of these difficulties in getting inpatient hospice units started in some hospitals, several different forms of hospice-like programs have emerged in hospitals. Sometimes they are actually called hospices, and other times they assume a variety of other names or titles.

For example, at St. Luke's Hospital Center in New York City, a group of hospital staff recognized how difficult it might be to start an inpatient hospice unit there, and as a result it proposed an entirely different form of hospital-based care of the dying—the symptom control team. This team was composed of clergy, nurses, physicians, social workers, and others interested in the care of the dying; its members served as consultants and sources of support and information to the regular staff providing care throughout the hospital. Patients were not collected in a single place or single ward within the hospital, a separate nursing staff was not utilized, and any appearance of a special unit was avoided. In general, the symptom control team did not take on the responsiblity for managing the actual patient care, although sometimes they would take charge of the home care arrangements after the patient had left the hospital.

In other hospitals, although staff members were not able to establish separate inpatient programs, they did arrange for the hospital to either sponsor its own home care program for dying patients or to affiliate with existing programs in the community. In these cases, a nursing staff member, who was either appointed by the hospital or who was assigned to work at the hospital by the community agency, served as the coordinator for the services to be provided to the patients at home. In this way, although the hospital might not itself have established an inpatient hospice unit, it could offer its patients hospice care at home after discharge, either through its own home care program or through a community program. (As a result of certain parts of the new Medicare hospice reimbursement legislation, this hospital-sponsored or hospital-affiliated type of hospice care has been given significant stimulus to develop further.)

The development of these three variants of hospital-based hospice programs in the United States and Canada gave hospital workers a variety of options to consider. Indeed, the appearance of these various hospital-based models of hospice care has made it possible for virtually every hospital to get involved with hospice care if it wishes to—and many hospitals have done so.

Community Models

Simultaneous to the development of these hospice programs in hospitals, a second and quite different stream of development was taking place in the communities outside hospitals, frequently under the leadership of people who had little or nothing to do with hospitals or sometimes even with health care in general. In the city of Bath, England, where the Dorothy House Foundation began its activities, and in Marin county in California, where the Hospice of Marin developed, new forms of community-based and community-sponsored hospice programs began to appear.

In general, the proponents of the initial community-based hospice programs established entirely new organizations to do the work that they had in mind, and in general these new organizations resembled social service agencies more than they did hospitals or clinics. The leadership was frequently drawn from the community at large, not from the health professions, and there was great interest in volunteer participation from persons in the community. There was comparatively little interest in financial matters, such as billing patients or insurance companies for service, and indeed, there was great interest in providing free service. Most of these new hospice programs spent a significant amount of time developing community support and interest, as well as identifying community needs and resources.

The range of direct services offered by these new community-based organizations varied widely, with a significant number of programs offering only volunteer-staffed, nonmedical and nonnursing, supportive kinds of services. In many of these programs, the leaders very often felt that they could not start out to actually provide much in the way of technical health care themselves, so they devoted their attention to those nontechnical personal support services that did not depend quite so much on the continuous availability of doctors, nurses, and other licensed professionals. In the beginning, these groups focused much more on psychological support groups, friendly visitor services, bereavement counseling, shopping and food-preparation assistance, transportation services, and the like (provided by their own workers), and they arranged for the more specialized services to be provided by other groups and organizations such as the local visiting nurse services.

After a while, a second type of community-based hospice program began to develop, this one within existing community agencies such as home health care programs or visiting nurse services. In general, these agencies would usually become involved initially by providing care for dying patients on an ad hoc, case-by-case basis, without any attempt to routinize or organize a special program or protocol of care for dying patients as a special group. As the concepts of care for the dying began to crystallize and as the identification of dying patients as a group needing special attention began to be better understood, many of these home care organizations developed hospice units or programs within the framework of their larger organizations, utilizing many of the already present staff and skills and frequently adding new ones as needed (such as bereavement counseling and counselors).

These second-generation community-based hospice programs differed from the first-generation ones in that they were seen from the beginning as professional health care agencies, operated by health care professionals and continuing a tradition and pattern of health care services that already existed. They generally had already established patterns of referral from physicians and hospitals in the community, and they spent more of their time and energies focusing on relations with the health care organizations and providers in the community than on the community itself.

In general, these second-generation community-based hospices were able to get organized more quickly and deliver a higher quality of technical services in a more efficient fashion than were the earlier type. These latter hospices were in agencies that had usually been in existence for some time, that knew where to find and hire professional personnel, that already had personnel practices and standards, and that had considerable experience in organizing and managing a work force. Also very important, they were frequently much more familiar with the intricacies of health insurance, both private and government, and knew better how to obtain whatever reimbursement might be available for providing care to the dying.

Definition and Standards

There are, then, at least six different forms that hospice programs take, all very similar in some respects but significantly different in others. After reviewing these varieties of organizational models, all of which either call themselves or are called by others *hospice,* it should be clear that hospice programs cannot be defined on the basis of their organizational form, their organizational sponsorship, or their location. Nor can hospices be defined on the basis of the services that they provide, because the package of services they provide varies widely among the organizational models and programs. Some hospices offer inpatient services through their own organization; others do not. Some hospices offer home care services through their own organizations; others obtain them from other organizations in the community.

How, then, does one define "hospice?" What is a hospice?

The National Hospice Organization (NHO) has faced this question and has developed a definition of hospice that clarifies matters considerably. NHO describes hospices as follows: "A hospice is a centrally administered *program* (emphasis author's) of palliative and supportive services which provides physical, psychological, social, and spiritual care for dying persons and their families. Services are provided by a medically supervised interdisciplinary team of professionals and volunteers. Hospice services are available in both the home and the inpatient setting. Home care is provided on a part-time, intermittent, regularly scheduled, and round-the-clock on-call basis. Bereavement services are available to the family. Admission to a hospice program of care is on the basis of patient and family need."[2]

There are several aspects of this definition that are worthy of note. First, NHO makes clear that hospice is a program, not a place or an organizational form. That is, hospice is an organized collection of services and is not defined by a physical structure or an organizational model of any kind. It is the content provided by the program that counts, not how or where the services are provided.

Second, it is implied that the hospice does not have to provide all the services itself, as long as they are available and coordinated in an organized fashion by the hospice. A hospice may purchase or obtain various services from health care providers, volunteers, community agencies, and physicians in the community, and then organize them into an integrated program of services.

What is the minimum basic set of services that must be included in a program of care for the dying that would allow it to be called a hospice? What are the organizational processes that must be present to link these individual services into an integrated program of care called hospice?

NHO has been interested in the question of definition and standards for hospice programs since its inception, and in 1979 it developed a set of standards for hospice care that describes the basic elements of an acceptable hospice program.[3] NHO revised these standards in 1981[4] and more recently has joined with the Joint Commission on Accreditation of Hospitals (JCAH) to develop an accreditation process for hospices based on these standards.[5,6] In order to put together these materials, the two groups drew upon their own past experience, as well as previous work by the American Nurses Association and the International Work Group on Death, Dying, and Bereavement.[7,8]

The following examination of those JCAH standards and draft accreditation criteria written by several hospice groups in California working with the California Medical Association[9] provides considerable insight into what the experts feel are the necessary elements of hospice programs.

Interdisciplinary Team

A hospice program should provide its care by means of an interdisciplinary team that includes at least medical direction, nursing services, social services, spiritual support, volunteer services, and bereavement counseling. There should be written policies and procedures stating the scope, documentation, and provision of team services, and the work of the inter-disciplinary team should be coordinated by a qualified health care professional who is acknowledged by all as the team leader. The interdisciplinary team members should conduct conferences regularly, and the results of their reviews and evaluations should be written in the patient/family record. The interdisciplinary team should receive continuing in-service training and education and should have access to organized programs of emotional support on a regular basis. The hospice program should have a medical director who, on the basis of training, experience, and interest, is knowledgeable about hospice services, the psychosocial care of patients and families, and the control of pain and other symptoms.

Patient-Family as the Single Unit of Care

In an acceptable hospice program, the patient and the patient's family are seen as the single unit of care. All of the hospice program's contacts with the patient must include appropriate contact with and involvement of the rest of the family unit as well. The patient and family must be assured that their beliefs will be respected and that the conduct of the patient's care will be in line with these beliefs. The patient will be the one to determine what the family unit will be, and it need not necessarily be limited to persons who are related to the patient by blood or by law.

Symptom Control

The care provided by an approved hospice program will be guided by a written plan for symptom control. This plan should include attention to both physical as well as emotional symptoms and should have a particular emphasis on the control of pain. Although control of pain should not be the only concern of hospice care, it is recognized that pain must be adequately controlled before any other hospice services can be maximally effective. As with all aspects of hospice care, symptom control should extend to the family members as well as the primary patient.

Continuum of Care

An acceptable hospice program provides a continuum of inpatient and home care services through an integrated administrative structure. These home care and inpatient services may be provided through various methods, depending upon the scope of services offered by the program itself, by local hospitals and health care agencies, and by resources in the community. No matter how they are provided, however, there should be a written set of agreements that govern the ways in which all the component parts will be brought together into a single pattern of care.

Most hospices will provide the home care themselves or will at least give a major emphasis to this portion of the hospice's total package of services. Home care service should include the ability to carry out initial assessments on the patient's and the family's needs for assistance and also the resources by which they can at least partially meet their own needs. The service should be available 24 hours a day, 7 days a week, and should be appropriately staffed to be able to deliver effective care to the patient/family at home up to the time of the patient's death. It should be equipped to continue some contact with the patient's family for a considerable time after the patient's death, if necessary.

An acceptable hospice program will provide specialized inpatient care for dying patients, either in a facility of its own or in another facility such as a hospital, nursing home, or freestanding hospice. When such services are not provided directly, there must be a written agreement with the organization or facility providing the services; this agreement must define the scope of contracted services and must ensure the continuity of contracted services with those provided directly by the program itself.

An approved hospice program must also have specific arrangements for providing bereavement services to the family members of its patients after the death of the patients. These services must be started with the family members while the patient is alive, in anticipation of death, and then must be continued for sufficient time after death to allow the family members to recover as fully as possible. As with the other services, bereavement services can be provided either by the hospice organization itself or by some other organization in the community, but it should most likely be provided by the hospice program.

Organization, Governance, and Management

For a hospice to be accepted as meeting the basic standards for such programs, it must have an organized governing body, or designated persons so functioning, which is responsible for establishing policy, maintaining high-quality patient-family care, and providing for management and planning for the hospice program. It must have a hospice program director appointed by the governing body or its appropriate administrative representative; this hospice program director is responsible for the operation of the organization. There must be adequate management and administrative staff, responsible to the program director, who can carry out the necessary administrative, financial, personnel, and other organizational functions to ensure the continued operation of the hospice.

These characteristics separate many of the current programs that care for dying patients from hospice programs. Many of the larger and better programs of comprehensive care for cancer patients offer the same services as hospices, yet they do not consider themselves hospices. They do not claim to be special terminal care programs or programs for the care of dying patients; they are caring for living patients and don't have a clearly identifiable separate program that could be called a hospice. If they should decide to be accredited or accepted as hospice programs, they would have to establish a more clearly defined program of care for the dying in order to be approved.

Finally, an acceptable hospice program must have a permanent management structure that ensures that the individual items of services will be provided in a well coordinated fashion. There must be a permanent organization that provides financial and management support to the entire hospice effort. There must be personnel structures that ensure that there will be adequate staff and that the staff will be handled in an orderly and stable fashion.

Utilization Review and Quality Control

An acceptable hospice program, like any other organized program of health services, must have a formal method for reviewing the appropriateness and the quality of the care being provided. Just as in any other health program, there must be written procedures for regularly carrying out organized review of patient care, with mechanisms established for taking action on deficiencies or problems that are discovered.

Commentary

The wide variety of organizational models for hospice programs and the wide variation among packages of services within the models deserve special attention for a number of reasons.

First, if it is presumed that all hospices are the same and public policy is developed that is appropriate to one type of hospice program, that policy may be entirely inappropriate for others. One form of licensure or accreditation that is appropriate for a hospital-based hospice program may not be appropriate for a community-based home care program, for example. One type of reimbursement formula for a program that provides all its hospice services itself, whether inpatient or home care, may not be entirely appropriate for another hospice program that merely provides a coordinating function and contracts with other community agencies for the bulk of the hospice services it offers.

Second, the development of public policy around one type or model of hospice program may encourage the development of that type of program or model but may also unwittingly or unintentionally discourage the development of others. Hospice care is still in its early stages of development and not everything has yet been learned about the best manner and method of delivering services. Nothing should be done that might inadvertently foreclose any potentially valuable new options or that might accidentally dampen the spirit of innovation and experimentation that has characterized hospice programs up to this point.

A third reason for avoiding the use of a single general all-inclusive model to describe hospice programs is that this might discourage the development of more specific descriptions of the various types of programs; it might discourage the careful identification of those specific characteristics of certain programs that make them more effective than others in certain circumstances and with certain patients. A premature lumping of all hospice programs into a single program description or a single policy might stop the process of analysis and development of new hospice variants — a process that is still greatly needed. Premature exclusion of some models would not only exclude those models; it would also exclude the patients those models are best at serving.

Summary

Merely calling an organization or a program a hospice doesn't make it one. There must be at least a minimal set of hospice services provided, there must be a clearly identifiable organization that is responsible for the total program of care, and there must be an intent to limit its attention and care to dying patients.

Although it is sometimes assumed that all hospice programs are similar, in fact the data that are available reveal remarkable differences between individual hospice programs. Not only are there several different organizational models of hospice in existence, but within the same types of hospice there are widely varied programs of service and methods of providing care.

Without more specific definitions and standards for hospice programs, it will be extremely difficult to plan for a community's future hospice needs, to evaluate the efficacy of hospice programs that come into existence, to license and accredit these programs in some rational fashion, and eventually to provide some solid financial support. More exact definitions and descriptions of hospice programs are a necessary precursor to the development of a rational public policy in this area.

References

1. Personal interviews, Apr.-May, 1979.
2. National Hospice Organization. *Standards of a Hospice Program of Care,* 6th revision. McLean, VA: NHO, 1979.
3. National Hospice Organization. *Standards,* 6th revision.
4. National Hospice Organization. *Revised Principles and Standards of Hospice Care.* Arlington, VA: NHO, 1981.

5. Joint Commission on Accreditation of Hospitals. *Hospice Standards Manual.* Chicago: JCAH, 1983.

6. Joint Commission on Accreditation of Hospitals. *Hospice Self-Assessment and Survey Guide.* Chicago: JCAH, 1983.

7. American Nurses Association. *Statement on Organized Care for the Terminally Ill and Their Families.* Washington, DC: ANA, 1979.

8. International Work Group on Death, Dying, and Bereavement. Assumptions and principles underlying standards for terminal care. *American Journal of Nursing.* 1979 Feb.

9. Hospice accreditation criteria, preliminary working draft. Mimeo, Bay Area Hospice Association (San Francisco)-California Medical Association-Southern California Hospice Association, San Francisco, 1982 June 18.

Chapter | **3**

Current Status of Hospice Programs

Paul R. Torrens, M.D., M.P.H.

What is the current status of hospice programs in the United States and elsewhere? How many programs are there, how are they organized, and what services do they offer to their patients?

Although exact data are difficult to obtain with regard to the specifics of hospice programs, it is possible to get some idea of the size and scope of the hospice movement by reviewing several recent surveys that have been carried out in this country, Canada, and Great Britain.

United States

There have been several surveys that have attempted to provide better insight into hospice program development in the United States. In 1979, the ELM Institute reviewed more than 250 applications from hospice programs to the U.S. Health Care Financing Administration for grant support and abstracted some general findings about the characteristics of these programs.[1] In 1979 and 1980, Robert Buckingham and Dale Lupu carried out a survey of a sample of the National Hospice Organization (NHO) membership and reported their findings and observations in 1982.[2] In 1981, the Joint Commission on Accreditation of Hospitals (JCAH) carried out a survey of all the hospice and hospice-like programs that it could identify;[3] parts of this survey were repeated in 1983-84.[4] Also in 1981, David Greer, Vincent Mor, and colleagues at Brown University reviewed the 26 hospice programs taking part in the National Hospice Study, a special research project sponsored by the Robert Wood Johnson Foundation, the

John A. Hartford Foundation, and the Health Care Financing Administration, and presented some preliminary observations from that review.[5] Further details from the National Hospice Study were presented in 1983.[6]

ELM Institute

The ELM Institute in 1979 reviewed the 259 applications received from hospice programs by the Health Care Financing Administration for a special hospice program grant solicitation. Of these 259 applications received, 83 had not then actually begun to deliver services and an additional 48 applications were either incomplete or in some way unsuitable for review, leaving 132 applications that could be reviewed.

In the review of these 132 applications, the ELM researchers developed a typology for identifying major hospice models; this typology was somewhat different from those previously discussed or used because it looked first at the predominant types of care offered rather than at the organization offering the care. This typology is listed below.

1. Home care services only; direct or contract services
2. Inpatient hospice care only; direct services
3. Home and inpatient care; direct or contract services
4. Home care services only; direct services as part of an organization (home health agency or hospital) providing other health care
5. Inpatient care only; direct services as part of an organization (hospital or nursing home) providing other health care
6. Home care and inpatient care; direct services as part of an organization providing other health care
7. Inpatient care in the form of a consultation team or consultation individual only; direct services as part of a hospital or nursing home
8. Home care in the form of a consultation team or consultation individual only

The ELM Institute determined that of the 132 organizations making application for the HCFA grant solicitation, 27 (20.4 percent) offered inpatient hospice care only, 5 (3.8 percent) offered both home and inpatient hospice care, 52 (39.4 percent) offered hospice home care as part of an organization (home health agency or hospital) providing a variety of other health care services, 4 (3 percent) offered inpatient hospice care only as part of an organization (hospital or nursing home) providing other inpatient care, 39 (29.5 percent) offered both home care and inpatient care as part of an organization providing other health care, 5 (3.8 percent) offered inpatient care in the form of only a consultation team or consultation individual as part of a hospital or nursing home, and none offered home care in the form of a consultation team or consultation individual only (see table 1, next page).

As can be seen by these results, the predominant model of service was the home care program of hospice service (79 of the total 132 organi-

Table 1. Service Models of Hospice Programs Applying for HCFA Grant Solicitation, January 1979

	Number	% of Total
Home care only	27	20.4
Inpatient hospice care only	0	0
Both home and inpatient care	5	3.8
Home care only, as part of an organization (home health agency or hospital) providing other health care	52	39.4
Inpatient care only, as part of an organization (hospital or nursing home) providing other health care	4	3.0
Both home and inpatient care, as part of an organization providing other kinds of health care	39	29.5
Inpatient care in the form of a consultation team or consultation individual only	5	3.8
Home care in the form of a consultation team or consultation individual only	0	0
Total	132	99.9

zations), with 27 of these being hospice organizations that provided no other types of health care and 52 being hospice programs located in agencies providing other kinds of care. Considerably fewer programs provided inpatient services of any kind (53 out of 132), 44 providing inpatient and outpatient care, 4 providing only inpatient care, and 5 providing only a consultation team or individual on an inpatient basis. Thus, in contrast to the Canadian and English situations in which inpatient units predominated, the more frequent model of service and of organization in the United States was outpatient home care.

It is interesting to note that almost all of the 132 hospice programs offered bereavement services of some kind (124 out of 132), but 8 programs (6 percent) did not, even though bereavement follow-up is considered almost the sine qua non of a hospice program. Only 72 percent of the programs stated that they had a designated medical director (whether full time or part time, paid staff or volunteer), and only 38 percent said that they utilized the services of physical therapists. Social workers were represented in 58 percent of the programs, and chaplains in 39 percent of the programs; registered nurses were included in the program staffing in 83 percent of the programs. It is noteworthy that less than 41 percent of the hospice programs utilized the services of volunteer health care professionals and less than 40 percent used the assistance of volunteer lay men and women.

Buckingham and Lupu

In 1979, Buckingham and Lupu carried out a survey on a sample of the 143 hospice members of the National Hospice Organization in 1978. In particular, they selected a subsample of 24 programs from those hospices that had delivered services for at least one year and that had served at least 100 patients since their development.

All of the hospices they studied were not-for-profit organizations, 10 of which were institutionally based (usually in a hospital), and the remainder, community based. All of the programs surveyed offered both home care and bereavement programs, but only 10 offered inpatient care. All but one of the 24 programs offered services 7 days a week and all but two offered them 24 hours a day. Two-thirds of the hospices augmented their own services through contracts with other agencies, 11 with visiting nurse associations and 11 with home health agencies.

The size of the programs ranged from a total admission of 40 a year in the smallest to 310 a year in the largest. Most of the hospices could not provide complete demographic information about their patients, but from what could be determined, the average patient was a white woman with a primary diagnosis of cancer, almost 60 years of age, and referred to the hospice by a physician. The average length of stay with the hospice program, whether as an inpatient or at home, was 47 days. In general, hospices did not seem to be operating at full capacity: for those hospices providing data, home care programs averaged 74 percent capacity; bereavement programs, 76 percent; and inpatient services, only 66 percent of estimated capacity.

In Buckingham and Lupu's study, only 21 of the 24 hospices were able to provide information on their total annual budget, and many programs could not give specific breakdowns of funding sources or budget allocations. Private sources (individuals and foundations) provided support to a majority of hospices. Third-party payers (private insurance carriers, Medicare, Medicaid, state and local government) were also prevalent, despite the lack of any significant national public program at the time of the survey to reimburse hospice services. Several hospices were recipients of federal grants that met a large portion of their operating costs.

Few hospices in Buckingham and Lupu's study reported the amount received from these sources, but for those that did so, the funding mix varied considerably from program to program. For example, the private donations received by the 16 hospices reporting their receipts ranged from $1,000 to $582,000 yearly, with an average of $70,000. Five programs reported yearly Medicare reimbursements ranging from $15,000 to $192,000, with an average of $117,400.

Fifty-seven percent of the 23 hospices providing information reported that they had experienced financial deficits during the previous year ranging from $5,000 in the smallest case to $240,000 in the largest. The most common explanation for these deficits was that bereavement services were generally not reimbursed by insurance or Medicare and that the home nursing visits to hospice patients took longer than other home visits, thereby costing more than the allowable reimbursement rate. Very few of the programs offering bereavement services charged the clients for these services.

Buckingham and Lupu made a rough estimate of per patient costs by calculating each program's total budget and dividing that by the total number of patients served each year. The crude nature of the data they had to deal with did not allow attempts to determine specific costs per patient day, per home visit, or per inpatient day or admission. The estimate for the costliest program was $43,338 per patient, whereas the mean cost per patient for all programs was $1,169. The median value was considerably less, $851, further emphasizing the great variability in costs among the programs. Buckingham and Lupu pointed out that these costs included only those services provided by the hospice program and did not include any costs incurred by the patients or their families outside the hospice program itself.

With regard to personnel and staffing, all but one of the hospices had at least one paid staff member; the average number of staff was 16.3 with a median of 9. All hospices employed secretaries and nurses in one capacity or another, but only 58 percent had a physician on staff, 62.5 percent had a social worker, 46 percent had a chaplain, 33 percent had a volunteer director, and only 16 percent had either an occupational therapist or a physical therapist.

All but one of the 24 hospices surveyed utilized volunteers in the program, with the size of the volunteer corps ranging from 3 in the smallest program to 400 in the largest; the average was 68 volunteers per site, with a median of 43. Twenty-three hospices had volunteers working in general home care, and almost 75 percent had volunteers working in bereavement, education, administration, and counseling. Of the 10 hospices offering inpatient services, only 6 had volunteers providing such services.

In general, Buckingham and Lupu's survey supported the general impressions of the other surveys that hospices were not regularly providing inpatient hospice care; only 10 of the 24 hospices in their survey offered inpatient care and only 4 more felt that it would be advantageous to have such services, even though they did not have such services at the time of the survey. In the same fashion, more than 40 percent of the hospices did not have a physician on staff, even though medical direction is felt to be an essential component of hospice programs.

Buckingham and Lupu's data also point out something that had previously been vaguely understood but not clearly recognized: a great amount of staff and volunteer time and effort in hospice programs is devoted to case management and not necessarily to the provision of direct services to individuals. As the authors point out, "Although hospice advocates recognize the need to coordinate existing community services in order to

avoid duplication, the hospice literature failed to suggest that this function would occupy so much time of hospice caregivers."

Joint Commission on Accreditation of Hospitals

In 1981, the Joint Commission on Accreditation of Hospitals carried out
a survey of hospices as part of a study of methods for possibly accrediting such programs in the future.[7] Although this survey focused primarily
on questions related to accreditation, it did provide some useful general
information concerning the services offered by hospice programs. Parts
of the survey were repeated in late 1983 and early 1984, providing some
updating on the 1981 information.[8]

In 1981 more than 800 hospice or hospice-like programs were identified and surveyed, of which 440 were classified as actually operational
at the time of the survey. By 1983-84, the total number of hospices had
risen to 1,429, of which 687 were actually providing care at the time of
the survey. A partial list of operating programs by state in 1981 and 1983-84
is given in table 2, next page.

In 1981, 48 percent of the hospices were hospital-owned, 32 percent
were owned by a community-based agency that provided only hospice care,
and 20 percent were owned by community agencies that also provided other
types of services, such as general home nursing care. By 1983-84, hospital-
owned hospices had dropped to 38 percent, independent hospice agencies
had risen to 38 percent, and hospices owned by community home health
agencies had remained at approximately 21 percent.

In the 1981 survey, it was found that home care only was provided
in 56 percent of the programs, home care and inpatient care was provided
in 36 percent, and inpatient care only was provided by 7 percent of the
programs. Thirty-two percent of the hospices in 1981 were not licensed
to give care in any capacity, and more than 40 percent were not accredited
by any accrediting body. Even in hospices that were accredited (60 percent), aspects of care that were specific to hospice were not surveyed as
part of the accreditation process; rather, hospice care programs were surveyed as part of accreditation surveys for hospitals, home health agencies, or long-term care facilities.

The 440 operational programs reviewed by JCAH in 1981 were generally new and small, with 51 percent becoming operational after January
1980, and with 75 percent of all programs admitting fewer than 100 patient-
family units in 1980. Only 2 percent of the programs admitted more than
250 patients in the year prior to the survey. The average monthly census
in 1981 (number of patient-family units per month per hospice, whether
inpatient or home care) was 17, with a current average caseload of 16
patient-family units and a current average bereavement caseload of 28.

In 1981, most of the programs (60 percent) had annual budgets of
under $75,000, with only 10 percent reporting budgets of more than

Table 2. Partial List of Hospice Programs by State, July 1981 and June 1984

	1981	1984		1981	1984
Alabama	5	12	Missouri	13	16
Alaska	—	2	Montana	5	5
Arizona	3	6	Nebraska	—	6
Arkansas	3	5	Nevada	1	1
California	67	95	New Hampshire	6	9
Colorado	6	17	New Jersey	17	31
Connecticut	1	11	New Mexico	3	6
Delaware	—	1	New York	17	20
District of			North Carolina	10	20
Columbia	2	2	North Dakota	1	1
Florida	14	17	Ohio	15	31
Georgia	7	13	Oklahoma	2	3
Hawaii	2	2	Oregon	9	7
Idaho	3	2	Pennsylvania	42	47
Illinois	20	48	Rhode Island	1	2
Indiana	11	12	South Carolina	3	5
Iowa	5	11	South Dakota	1	1
Kansas	11	8	Tennessee	5	16
Kentucky	11	9	Texas	—	15
Louisiana	3	4	Utah	—	6
Maine	—	21	Vermont	6	5
Maryland	9	16	Virginia	4	10
Massachusetts	19	37	Washington	15	17
Michigan	—	19	West Virginia	—	6
Minnesota	20	13	Wisconsin	—	20
Mississippi	3	2	Wyoming	—	1
Totals				401	692

Sources: Falknor, P., and Kugler, D. JCAH hospice project, interim report: Phase I. Mimeo, Joint Commission on Accreditation of Hospitals, Chicago, 1981 July; Joint Commission on Accreditation of Hospitals. JCAH hospice provider profile. Mimeo, JCAH, Chicago, 1984 June.

$300,000. In about half of the programs, foundation and donation monies accounted for more than 40 percent of the budget. In general, most of the programs seemed to offer all of the expected hospice services, with the exception of homemaker services and respite care, that is, relief for family caregivers for a short period of time.

As part of the 1981 JCAH survey, in-depth site visits were made to 17 hospice programs of various kinds, and a number of important subjective impressions were formed. All 17 programs were under some form of medical direction, either full-time or, more often, part-time and volunteer. There were usually a number of mechanisms established for involving the patient's attending physician in the activities of the hospice program. Pain and symptom control were central and primary aspects of all 17 programs, and psychosocial, spiritual, and financial counseling were a part of most programs. Services were always directed towards the patient and the family as a single unit, the family being defined according to the patient's wishes. Some form of contact or communication was always available 24 hours a day, 7 days a week, although the intensity of service and support available varied considerably. Interestingly enough, the on-call service seemed to be very infrequently utilized by the patients and their families, perhaps because of the conscientious preparation of patients and families for what to anticipate on their return home.

All of the hospice programs utilized volunteers in some aspects of the program, but their actual roles varied widely from routine chores of a clerical and administrative nature to a more client-focused service role of direct assistance. Bereavement programs for family members were a part of all the 17 hospice programs visited, but the degree of sophistication and the level of intensity of services varied considerably.

Most of the home care hospice programs in 1981 had referral mechanisms to hospitals, but in almost all instances these hospitals did not have any special hospice care programs or provisions of their own. Hospice staff usually had permission to follow their patients in these hospitals, in order to provide continuity of care, psychosocial support, and assistance to the hospital staff in pain and symptom control as well as in discharge planning.

National Hospice Study

In 1980, Greer, Mor, and colleagues at Brown University began a major study of hospice programs, the National Hospice Study, in order to determine more accurately the costs of providing hospice care, the quality and effectiveness of the care being provided, and the potential impact of Medicare and Medicaid financing on hospice programs. In the process of carrying out this study, the researchers documented many characteristics of the 40 hospices included in the study (26 demonstration hospices and 14 control or nondemonstration hospices), as well as much information about the patients currently being served by them.[9,10]

Forty-seven percent of the hospices were found to be hospital-based or hospital-affiliated, 23 percent were affiliated with home health agencies, and 30 percent were freestanding or independent, that is, not affiliated with an existing health care provider. It was noted that there were significant variations among the hospices themselves and also among the classes of hospices, with the hospital-based hospices seeming to have those patients who were the sickest and who had fewer social supports outside the hospital.

Slightly more than half the patients in the National Hospice Study were female (53.3 percent), 61 percent were married, and slightly fewer than a quarter (23.8 percent) were widowed. Fewer than 10 percent were nonwhite, fewer than one-third were Catholic, more than one-third were Protestant, and for one-third a religious affiliation could not be determined. More than 65 percent of the patients were over 65 years of age, and only about 1 percent were less than 35 years of age. Although not an affluent population, nearly 20 percent had a family income of $20,000 or more.

The most common living arrangement (58 percent) was a patient living with a spouse; somewhat fewer patients lived with other family members, and fewer than 10 percent lived alone. Most of the hospices surveyed by Greer and Mor either required or preferred that patients have a person designated as the primary caregiver who could assist in the provision of care in the home, so it was no surprise in this study to find that most patients did have such a person living with them. In more than 55 percent of the cases, the primary caregiver was the patient's spouse, but in 15 percent of the cases it was someone actually living outside the patient's household.

In the hospices studied, cancer patients constituted approximately 90 percent of all patients, although certain participating hospices served more than 20 percent of patients whose diagnoses were other than cancer. Analyses of data on the noncancer patients revealed that they had significantly longer stays in hospice and that they appeared to use almost twice as many hours of homemaker and nursing services at home as the cancer patients.

The distribution of cancer types among the hospice patients was typical of the national figures for cancer prevalence, with cancer of the lung being the most prevalent, followed by cancer of the colon, breast, and prostate. As might be expected, the hospice patients were found to be severely ill and functionally limited, with fewer than 20 percent being able to walk alone on admission, nearly 19 percent having a urinary catheter in place, and 20 percent requiring oxygen on admission. Patients admitted to the hospital-based hospices were considerably sicker on admission than those patients admitted to home health agency hospices.

In the study, patients were referred to the hospice programs from a variety of sources. In hospital-based hospices and in independent or freestanding hospices, the most common primary referral source was a physician; in home health agency hospices, the primary referral sources were discharge planners in hospitals. Family members and friends were twice as likely to be the primary referral source in freestanding hospices, but the patient was almost never the primary referrer to any of the programs.

It found that 49 percent of the patients originally admitted to a hospice program died at home. However, this figure varied considerably among the types of hospices, with fewer than 20 percent of the hospital-based hospice patients dying at home as compared to more than 60 percent of the home care hospice patients. In general, hospice patients were found to be more severely ill on admission than had originally been anticipated, with 40 percent of the patients dying within the first three to four weeks after admission.

The National Hospice Study data also indicated significant differences among patient populations among the various types of hospices, differences mostly in severity of illness at the time of admission and in the ability to remain home until death but also in the diagnostic mix of the cancers themselves. The researchers have pointed out the extreme caution that must be used in comparing various aspects of hospice work or, indeed, in comparing hospices to more traditional forms of care. Unless there is some standardization for severity of illness in patients served, comparisons across hospice types or of hospice care and traditional care probably are not valid.

Canada

In late 1981 and early 1982, a survey of palliative care programs in Canada was undertaken by the Palliative Care Foundation in Toronto.[11] In many ways, the survey was similar to that undertaken by the Joint Commission on Accreditation of Hospitals in the United States, in that the surveyors actively worked to identify all hospice or hospice-like programs in Canada by querying knowledgeable persons in Canada and all hospitals in every province.

The survey showed that there were 64 existing palliative care programs in Canada, with a further 18 programs or services that were to be implemented within 12 months of the survey. An additional 25 hospitals stated that, even though they did not have formal programs of palliative care, they felt that they followed the general philosophy of palliative care in their present programs and that they included the usual hospice-component services in their regular array of services. An additional 8 hospitals indicated a definite intention to implement a service in the near future, the details of which were currently being developed. This means that in Canada at the time of the survey, there were 64 existing palliative care programs of one kind or another, there were an additional 25 programs that were considered by their sponsoring hospitals to have met the usual criteria for hospice programs although they were not labeled as such, and there were an additional 26 programs planned to begin sometime in the future.

These services or programs varied considerably in size, however, ranging from those in several large teaching hospitals with a complete ward or wards of designated beds for hospice patients to those services or programs operated by a single person. Of the 56 programs for which staffing details were available, 35 (62.5 percent) were staffed by multidisciplinary teams including at least one physician and one nurse, plus some other personnel such as social workers, chaplains, volunteers, and physiotherapists. Of the other 21 programs for which staffing information was available, 14 (25 percent) did not include a physician, and 3 of these 14 (5 percent) did not include either a physician or a nurse; a further 3 of these 14 (5 percent) were staffed by a single nurse. Two services consisted of a single physician only, and 5 did not have any specified staffing but drew on the general staff complement of the hospital.

With regard to the services offered by the individual programs, 20 (34.5 percent) of the 58 programs for which the information was available had inpatient beds specifically designated for their patients, whereas 38 (63.5 percent) used whatever beds were available scattered throughout the hospital. Eighteen (31 percent) of the 58 programs provided only inpatient services, and the remaining 40 programs (69 percent) provided home care as well as inpatient services. In all, a total of 241 hospital beds specifically designated for palliative care patients could be identified in all hospitals throughout Canada; the number of nondesignated beds, used intermittently, could not be documented.

Virtually all the palliative care programs in Canada included symptom control services and counseling for both patients and families before death. Only 75 percent of the services, however, included counseling for the family after the death of the patient. Religious counseling was included to a high degree (79 percent of all programs), as was staff education (80 percent). A few respondents also mentioned additional services such as music therapy, dietetic services and dietary counseling, and clinical pharmacy services.

In general, the majority of the formally organized existing programs (32 out of 59 services, or 54 percent) were located in hospitals with more than 300 beds; of these 32, 14 services (24 percent of the total 59) were located in general teaching hospitals. Of the informal palliative care services (that is, those hospitals that believed they were providing care that followed the usual model of hospice programs), the great majority were located in small hospitals and, particularly, small hospitals in the western prairie provinces.

Overall, there were many more palliative care programs in Canada than had originally been suspected, but the level of intensity of services varied widely among the programs; for at least one-third of the programs, it hardly seemed appropriate to call them programs at all, since the staffing was so low (or even nonexistent). There was a heavy preponderance of hospital sponsorship, with the great majority of programs either having their origins in hospitals or having strong hospital support or encouragement. There was also a growing interest in starting new hospice programs, as evidenced by the 26 hospitals planning new programs.

Great Britain

In January 1980, Barry Lunt conducted a detailed survey of hospice programs in England, Scotland, and Wales* and found that there were 63 separate hospice programs providing services.[12-15] These 63 programs provided 55 inpatient units, 23 home care services, and 5 hospital support (symptom control) teams in a variety of combinations.

The majority of these 63 programs (two-thirds) offered only an inpatient service, and 5 of these programs offered only a home-care service. The remaining programs (one-third) offered both inpatient and outpatient services to their patients. Hospital support (symptom control) teams were offered by programs that also offered either inpatient or outpatient service as well.

Twenty-eight of the 63 programs were operated by the National Health Service. The Marie Curie Memorial Foundation and the Sue Ryder Foundation, two private charities interested in terminal care, operated 10 and 4 programs, respectively. Almost all of the other services throughout Great Britain were run as small, independent charities.

Different types of services were provided by the different programs in Great Britain. The Marie Curie homes, the private nursing homes, and most of the Sue Ryder homes were inpatient units only, whereas many of the National Health Service and local charity services provided a combination of inpatient and home care.

There were wide regional variations in the level of provision of terminal care, with the southeast regions of Great Britain generally better off in terms of both inpatient units and home care services. Growth has been rapid in Great Britain, with almost all the home care services and hospital support teams developing between 1975 and the time of the study in 1980; the number of inpatient units more than doubled during that period.

The most common size of inpatient units in Great Britain was 21 to 30 beds, although the range was wide. Most of the inpatient units operated by the National Health Service had been built expressly for use as hospice programs, whereas most of the privately operated programs used facilities that had been converted from another purpose. Slightly more than half of the inpatient units were situated on their own grounds at a distance from any hospital, and slightly less than half were situated within a hospital or at least on the grounds of a hospital. Almost all of the programs located on their own grounds were operated by private charities, whereas most of the programs located on the grounds of hospitals were operated by the National Health Service.

---

*Most of the material in this section is drawn, with permission, from the summary section of Lunt's report on his work.

The capital costs of constructing the units in the National Health Service were provided by a private charity, the National Society for Cancer Relief. The non-NHS services were generally funded from several sources, including the National Society for Cancer Relief, the National Health Service, and a variety of private foundations. The arrangements for obtaining operating costs of all the units were somewhat complicated, with about half the units receiving funding from several sources. The National Health Service generally provided all of the costs for all of its own units and a significant proportion of the operating costs for many of the private units.

Twenty-two of the 55 inpatient units had definite catchment areas to which they tried to limit their patients; these varied in size from 17,000 to 5 million, with a median of 500,000 total population. The level of provision of inpatient beds varied from 6 to 150 terminal-care beds per million population. None of those units providing fewer than 20 beds per million was thought to satisfy its area's requirements. Of those that were thought to give a satisfactory level of coverage, the median level was 44 beds per million population. (These estimates were based on subjective opinions obtained from hospice workers throughout Great Britain and should be interpreted with care.)

The majority of the programs relied on outside physicians to provide medical supervision as needed, with only 10 units having a full-time medical director or consultant. Seventeen more had part-time consultants, and the rest relied on physicians to the community. Slightly more than half the units had some sort of social work input, although this varied greatly in its extent. Occupational therapy and physiotherapy followed similar patterns. Less than half the units provided bereavement follow-up, and these were mostly units that had social workers on their staff.

The mean number of admissions per bed per year was 11.4 for the units within the National Health Service, 10.2 for the units run by local independent charities, 7.1 admissions per bed per year in the Sue Ryder homes, and 5.9 in the Marie Curie Foundation homes. The average length of stay in these inpatient units was 21.3 days for the NHS programs, 31.2 days for the independent charity programs, and 26.7 days for the Sue Ryder homes. The Marie Curie Foundation homes were unable to provide length-of-stay data.

Of the 23 home care services in Great Britain, 18 were associated with inpatient units of one kind or another, and 5 operated independently of an inpatient specialist unit. Most of the home care services had a single source of support for operating costs, but, interestingly enough, this source of support was often not the organization or body that actually ran the program itself. Many of the home care programs in the National Health Service, for example, were supported by grants from the National Society for Cancer Relief, and many of the home care services operated by private charities were supported by grants from the National Health Service.

The home care nurses provided the usual array of direct services to individual patients in their programs. They also provided advice to general practitioners and district public health nurses, counseling to patients and families, and bereavement follow-up services to families.

Nearly all of the home care services had defined catchment areas, mostly adhered to, that ranged from 24,000 people to 2 million. The scale of provision per full-time-equivalent nurse varied from 30,000 to 500,000 population. The ideal size of the catchment was thought to be limited by the distance the nurses had to travel; the maximum distance recommended averaged 12 miles, less in urban areas and more in rural.

Current work load varied widely, with a median of 15 patients per full-time nurse; this figure was higher in the home care programs operated by the National Health Service and lower in the programs operated by the private charities. The annual work load also showed great variations among the different home care programs, with a median of 64 new patients per full-time nurse per year being the average in the National Health Service programs and 45 new patients per full-time nurse per year in the private charity programs.

Despite the reputations of St. Christopher's, St. Joseph's, and others for providing extensive and comprehensive care, the majority of hospice programs in Great Britain seem to be focused on providing inpatient care, frequently in freestanding units located at some distance from hospitals.

This opinion, however, must be tempered by the realization that there is already a much wider array of community services provided to patients and their families in their homes in Great Britain than there is in the United States and Canada, as has been pointed out by Smith and Granbois.[16] Great Britain has an extensive system of district and community nursing services, usually well integrated with an extensive system of family practice physicians, most of whom still make home visits to their patients. These two systems, working together and providing attention to patients in their own homes, actually have reduced the need for a more comprehensive program of hospice care in Great Britain. Such a comprehensive program might be thought necessary in North America, however, because of our somewhat fragmented and noncomprehensive system of community health and home care services.

Summary

In retrospect, what general statements can be made, what general conclusions can be drawn from this diverse collection of data from various parts of the world? What useful and instructive lessons can be learned from reviewing the surveys that have thus far been carried out?

It should first be noted that although there is an increasing wealth of information about the actual *numbers* of hospice programs that are in existence, there is actually very little detailed information about the intensity of services those hospice programs provide and, more important, very little information about the impact on the patients served. There still is actually very little information available on the numbers of patients being served per year, and there is virtually no information about the numbers and kinds of patients *not* being served (that is, the unmet need for hospice care in our communities).

Of the existing programs themselves, the generalization could be made that programs in England are more likely to be predominantly inpatient in nature and located either in freestanding hospices or in hospital-operated specialist units. The inpatient units are generally larger than similar units in Canada or the United States and are generally quite substantial operations.

By contrast, the palliative care programs in Canada are hospital-based or hospital-sponsored, and there are virtually no freestanding hospices and relatively few community-based hospice programs. The hospital-sponsored palliative care programs in Canada may be rather sizeable operations depending on their location, but they may also be quite small programs with no actual inpatient beds of their own and virtually no permanent or even part-time staff.

Hospice programs in the United States are primarily home care in nature and orientation, even though their sponsorship is equally divided between hospitals and community agencies of one kind or another. They are still generally small programs, serving comparatively small numbers of patients with few permanent staff members. They are relatively new, having come into existence only in the past few years, and they all seem to have significant financial problems. Both the array of services offered and the intensity of these services vary widely from one program to another, so that it is very difficult to compare the services of one program with those of another.

With regard to the patients themselves in United States hospice programs, almost all have cancer; most are female, more than 65 years of age, nonminority, and with a slightly higher income than the national average. Recent work has suggested that patients in different types of hospices vary, with some degree of either patient selection or program selection taking place; patients in hospital-based hospice programs tend to be sicker, to need more care, and to have less home support from caregivers than do patients in community-based hospice programs. Until more is known about this difference in patient subpopulations among various kinds of hospices and between hospices and traditional programs of care, comparisons of results and of financial requirements should be made cautiously, if at all.

For the present, the details of hospice care in the United States and Canada can only be discussed in general terms, as there are no uniform data-collecting systems in place yet and little standardization of terms and procedures. With the development of the Medicare hospice benefits, more improved data about the hospices themselves, the patients they serve, and the utilization of those services will become more readily available. It will be important for all people interested in hospice care to analyze these data carefully and to begin to plan the future of the hospices of this country on the basis of that information. Also, over the years, the hospice programs themselves and the National Hospice Organization will have to design and implement new uniform data sets that more accurately describe what hospices are doing and how they are doing it, so that the progress of hospice care can be more expertly guided and supported by those in public policy positions.

References

1. Wilson, D. C., English, D. J., and Research Staff of ELM Institute. *An assessment of the existing staffing patterns and personnel required in a hospice to deliver interdisciplinary patient care and the problems related to delivering humanistic care to hospice patients.* (Prepared under DHEW Contract No. HRA 232-79-0082.) Hyattsville, MD: Bureau of Health Professions, Health Resources Administration, 1980 July.

2. Buckingham, R. W., and Lupu, D. A comparative study of hospice services in the United States. *American Journal of Public Health.* 1982 May. 72(5):455-63.

3. Falknor, P., and Kugler, D. JCAH hospice project, interim report: Phase I. Mimeo, Joint Commission on Accreditation of Hospitals, Chicago, 1981 July.

4. Joint Commission on Accreditation of Hospitals. JCAH hospice provider profile. Mimeo, JCAH, Chicago, 1984 June 20.

5. Greer, D., Mor, V., and others. Evaluating the impact of hospice care: The National Hospice Study design. Mimeo, presented at 109th annual meeting, American Public Health Association, Los Angeles, 1981 Nov. 4.

6. Mor, V., and Birnbaum, H. Medicare legislation for hospice care: Implications of National Hospice Study data. *Health Affairs.* 1983 Summer. 2(2):80-90.

7. Falknor and Kugler.

8. Joint Commission on Accreditation of Hospitals.

9. Greer, Mor, and others.

10. Mor and Birnbaum.

11. Southall, H. A survey of palliative care programmes and services in Canada. Mimeo, Palliative Care Foundation, Toronto, 1982 Dec.

12. Lunt, B. Terminal cancer care: Specialist services available in Great Britain in 1980. Survey report, Wessex Regional Cancer Organization and the University of Southampton, 1981 Mar.

13. Taylor, H. *The Hospice Movement in Britain: Its Role and Its Future.* London: Centre for Policy on Aging, 1983.

14. Lunt, B. Terminal care services in Great Britain: The current picture and future developments. St. Christopher's Hospice, Sydenham, England, 1983.

15. Lunt, B., and Hillier, R. Terminal care: Present services and future priorities. *British Medical Journal.* 1981 Aug. 283:595-98.

16. Smith, D., and Granbois, J. The American way of hospice. *Hastings Center Report.* 1982 Apr.

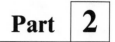

Issues in Hospice Care in the United States

Chapter 4

Which Dying Patients Should Hospices Serve?

Paul R. Torrens, M.D., M.P.H.

Everyone who has heard of hospice programs knows that they are supposed to care for the dying. Very few, however, ask the important question *"Which* dying patients should they serve?" Although this may seem to be a strange and almost ludicrous question, it is in fact a very central policy question that must be addressed directly by all who are interested in the development of hospice programs in the future.

Difficult Death versus Dying Patients

When Cicely Saunders, M.D., and her early colleagues in England began their work in the late 1950s and early 1960s, they were appalled at the level of unmet needs among dying patients in hospitals. There was inadequate control of pain, insufficient psychological support for patients and families, and general unavailability of adequate physical surroundings in which the dying process could unfold at its own pace and in a generally supportive atmosphere.

Implicit in their early work was the assumption that a considerable number of patients were dying difficult deaths and that a new form of care was needed for them, a form of care that would respond more appropriately to the needs of the patients and their families and that would more appropriately handle those special problems with which hospitals simply could not cope. There was an assumption that, even at its best, the average acute care general hospital was not able to meet the needs of many of its patients and that a new form of care was needed.

The solution in England was the development of the specialized unit to handle particular problems of dying patients. This development followed a pattern that had already been well established in England and elsewhere, the establishment of a special unit to provide care for particularly complex and hard-to-manage illness. Indeed, the creation of these specialized units was often seen as a way to draw attention to a particular problem and to obtain special funding and financial support that might otherwise not be available.

As the years progressed, however, and as the early hospice experience began to be more widely reviewed and enthusiastically admired, a rather rapid (and generally unrecognized) change began to take place with regard to the objectives of hospice programs, both in England and, more strongly, in the United States. Whereas previously the focus of hospice programs' efforts had been on the difficult deaths of patients whose needs could not be met in general hospitals, gradually the emphasis began to move more broadly towards *all* dying patients, regardless of whether their death seemed to be difficult or not. In many ways, it began to be assumed that *all* deaths were difficult and had a right to the extraordinarily sensitive kind of care provided in hospices.

Indeed, in the United States almost from the very beginning of the hospice movement, the idea of hospice was that of a general care, community-based program, not that of a specialized inpatient referral unit to which only the patients with unmanageable or difficult medical problems were sent. It seemed to be the opinion that any dying patient should have the benefit of a hospice program, even if the needs of that patient could have been handled in a general hospital. It was thought that the hospice program could clearly do the job better, so therefore all dying patients should have access to one, regardless of whether the program might duplicate hospital services.

In retrospect, it seems that this question has been viewed too briefly and without real understanding of the implications, if indeed it has been reviewed at all. On the one hand, if it is agreed that hospice programs should really be specialized "backup" units that are called into play only when it is obvious that standard programs of care are not capable of handling the challenge, the model of hospice that then develops will reflect this decision. This kind of hospice unit will generally be fewer in number, will have extensive inpatient facilities, and will have rather high-powered specialist teams who work in hospice programs and nowhere else. The units will be referral centers of a specialized nature, will conduct research and advanced teaching, and will generally represent the most advanced state of the art of hospice care.

On the other hand, if it is agreed that hospice care should be provided to *all* dying patients and that the mere fact of a terminal illness will call into play a hospice program's services, then a quite different model of hospice will result. In this model, there will be a much greater number of programs, spread more broadly throughout the community and, indeed, the country. They will be more general in nature and less intensely specialist, and they will offer more outpatient and in-home services than inpatient and special care unit services. The staff will be more generally trained and may not even limit their professional activities just to hospice patients. They may not even consider themselves specialists in the care of the dying, but rather see themselves as providing good medical or nursing care to a somewhat special population. In these more general programs, most certainly less research will be conducted, and probably less advanced education and training will be carried out. By and large, these programs will be the equivalent of the small, more general community hospital, whereas the previous programs will correspond to the most specialized tertiary hospital.

At the present time, most hospice programs try to fulfill both functions, that is, serve both as a unit of special competence for handling the difficult deaths, as well as a more general unit of total support for patients requiring less complicated care. There may, however, be some logic in reviewing this situation again in light of the accumulated experience across the country and in light of data (such as that of David Greer and Vincent Mor discussed in chapter 3) that show some significant differences in the patient populations served by institution-based hospice programs and community-based ones.

What will most probably emerge will be a full spectrum of hospice programs that range from the most general, community-based, nonspecialized ones that provide a broad base of care to all dying patients, on through several more specialized variations, and finally reaching a small number of highly specialized referral units where vigorous research and teaching are actively carried on.

The challenge for each individual hospice unit and the accompanying challenge to those involved in public policy for hospices will be to determine where exactly on the spectrum of specialization each unit sits and, more important, how many units of each kind this country will need in the future. The important question of the future may possibly no longer be "Which dying patients should hospices serve?" Instead, it may well be "Which dying patients should be served by which hospices?"

Cancer versus Noncancer Deaths

In all the surveys of hospice programs and the patients they serve, it is repeatedly shown that 90 to 95 percent of the patients are dying from cancer. Indeed, these same surveys often highlight the fact that many hospice programs will not take on patients unless there is a clear indication that death is relatively near, usually no further away than three to six months from the time of referral. Hospice programs do not take care of dying patients; they take care of patients dying with cancer who will probably die in a relatively short period of time.

It is interesting to note that when Saunders opened St. Christopher's Hospice in 1967, at least 10 percent of its ward beds were designated for patients with advanced neurological diseases. Speaking on the occasion of the 13th anniversary of the opening of St. Christopher's, Saunders and her colleagues described their experience in taking care of more than 100 patients with advanced motor neuron disease (amyotrophic lateral sclerosis), a chronic progressive neurological condition that eventually leads to a difficult death, but one whose progress is certainly not rapid or predictable with regard to time. Saunders and her colleagues stressed the importance of this experience for the staff of the hospice.[1,2]

Different program models will emerge, depending on the way in which individual programs answer the question "Which dying patients should hospices serve?" On the one hand, if programs review the question in the light of the issues raised above and reaffirm their commitment to the care of patients dying with cancer, one type of program will emerge. This program will be specific in its objectives and organization, will be able to train its staff in the particular needs of cancer patients, and will be able to deliver a very specific set of services of high quality. There will be a fairly rapid turnover of patients, there will be a clear identification of the program's purposes in the minds of the public and the staff, and there will generally be more enthusiasm for the program and its activities. It will also care for only a portion of a community's dying patients.

On the other hand, if the staff of an individual program reviews this question and decides to expand its effort by caring for patients dying of various conditions and at varying speeds, a different type of program model will emerge. It will be more diffuse in purpose and will be seen less clearly by the community and by its own staff. It will have to develop a broader range of services and capabilities and will not be able to provide its patients and staff with prepackaged programs for accomplishing certain objectives. The turnover of patients will be less rapid and certainly less predictable and the measurement of outcomes and the attainment of financial support more difficult. In general, the program will look less like the hospice program of the present and more like a general service community agency, whether it be an inpatient unit or a home care program.

Patients with Primary Caregivers versus Patients Without

A recent paper by Butterfield-Picard and Magno described what they call the "Catch-22 of hospice primary caregiver requirements."[3] Although the title may sound somewhat frivolous, the phenomenon they discuss certainly is not.

In their article, they point out that a recent Department of Health and Human Services (DHHS) survey of hospices showed that 67 percent required that a potential patient have a primary caregiver available at home as a condition for admission.[4] The primary caregiver could be either a family member or a friend who lives with the patient and who is available to the patient at least 19 hours a day. Hospices with a requirement for a primary caregiver in attendance believe that hospice care cannot be carried out adequately or safely without the presence of this intermediary.

As Butterfield-Picard and Magno point out, however, this requirement simply does not correspond to the realities of life for potential hospice patients in the United States today. Almost 60 percent of present American hospice patients are over 65 years of age, and the majority are women. In this population of women over the age of 65, unfortunately, more than 65 percent live alone, even though some familial ties may still exist.

In other words, the population that would ordinarily be most likely to utilize hospice programs and perhaps the one most likely to benefit from their services is specifically prevented from using those hospice services by reason of their isolation and lack of a primary caregiver. Butterfield-Picard and Magno quote officials of DHHS who say, "If a solution to this difficult situation is not found, an important segment of the population will be denied hospice services."

It is certainly true that good hospice care is easier to give when there is a primary caregiver in the home with whom the hospice program can work; it does make the work of the hospice team more effective and also more efficient. However, this does not mean that it is impossible to give good hospice care if there is no primary caregiver available; it only means that it is more difficult. Hospice programs will have to examine their policies in this regard and individually decide whether they want to exclude the most needy portion of the dying population because it is more difficult to provide care to them.

'Heavy-Care' Patients versus 'Light-Care' Patients

There is a broad spectrum of utilization of services among patients in hospices. Some patients admitted to a hospice require comparatively little in the way of direct nursing care or special support services; together with their families and friends, they seem to cope rather well, do not pose serious management dilemmas, and utilize relatively little in the way of program resources.

Most hospice programs, however, have seen patients who have utilized great amounts of program staff time and resources, who are constantly on the verge of being readmitted to the hospital, and whose condition calls for a heavy program of services and care.

This wide range should not come as a surprise, as it is generally the same in all organized health care programs. The surprise is probably that it has taken us so long to recognize that not all dying patients are the same in their requirements for services and that programs will have to learn better to appraise patients' real needs for service and the hospice program's real ability to meet those needs.

It may be that, in the future, hospice programs or hospice experts of one kind or another will be better able to categorize the severity of the patient's illness in terms of utilization of resources and will be better able to fit this information into planning for the patients and the program itself. It may be that in the future, for example, a community-based home care hospice will realize that it can take on no more than six heavy-care patients in its case load at the same time without unduly overburdening the staff and the program. If a seventh heavy-care patient needs admission, the hospice program may then need to take on extra staff to care for that patient, or it may wish to refer the patient to another program if one is available. Indeed, if there is no other hospice program available to share the load, the hospice program may advise the patient's physician to keep the patient in the hospital a bit longer, until the hospice program's case load of heavy-care patients becomes somewhat lighter.

It may also be useful in the future to better categorize patients' need for and utilization of services, in order to ensure that insurance payments and reimbursement levels are appropriate for the level of care given. For example, two hospice programs may look exactly alike in all respects except that one program has a much greater case load of heavy-care patients than the other. In comparing the results of these two programs and in setting reimbursement levels for the two, it would be important to know these details so that more accurate and appropriate comparisons of effect can be made and the program with the case load requiring greater services can receive a higher level of financing.

Finally, there may be some hospice programs that may wish to limit their particular services to one part of the spectrum of patients and not work with all dying patients. An individual hospice program, particularly one that is based within a hospital or an institutional setting, may wish to concentrate on the sicker patients, those requiring a heavier pattern of patient care services. The rationale may be, "There are already programs that exist to care for the less difficult patients who use fewer services. Let's concentrate our efforts on the patients who can't get our level of care from any other hospice program."

In the same vein, a community-based program may recognize the limitations of its resources and may not want to oversell its services to patients and families, promising them something it cannot deliver. This program may say, "We can care for patients with this particular level of need, but if it seems that they are going to need a lot more than that, perhaps we had better arrange for them to obtain their hospice care somewhere else."

At the present time, there are no good or easy measures to determine whether a particular patient is going to require a heavy pattern of care or a light one. Indeed, it may be impossible to ever do so at all. However, every hospice program and every person involved with hospice programs and policy should realize that not all hospice patients are the same with regard to the level of their need for service.

Middle-Class versus Minority and Disadvantaged Patients

Looking again at reports of patients served by hospice programs, it becomes increasingly clear that hospices are now basically a middle-class phenomenon. The predominant patients are female, white, and have a family in attendance. Indeed, in many cases the hospice programs insist that potential patients have a home to return to and a family to support them when they return home.

The problem, unfortunately, is that there are many dying patients who do not fit easily into this comfortable general plan, who are not middle class, who do not have private health insurance or a private physician, and who do not have a home or a family. Frequently, these patients are receiving their care in city or county hospitals in which there are no hospices available and in which referral patterns to outside hospices simply are not known. For example, in Los Angeles County (where this author resides), the county government operates four large, acute care general teaching hospitals and cares for large numbers of patients with cancer; there were no hospice or palliative care programs of a formal nature in any of these hospitals as of early 1983.

Frequently, too, these patients have serious problems with alcohol and other related conditions that interfere with their potential adjustment to a hospice regimen. They frequently come into the hospital for cancer care at a somewhat later stage in the disease, so that the staff is unable to prepare for the dying process as well as it might.

This relative underrepresentation of lower socioeconomic and minority patients is not unique to hospices by any means. The same pattern of underrepresentation seems to hold true for nursing homes, in which the same predominance of white women of middle-class background is seen. The reason for this pattern in nursing homes is not any better understood than it is for hospice programs, but it seems to be related to the prior availability of a private physician, access to a voluntary not-for-profit (or at least, nongovernment) hospital, and the presence of a family that is at least interested in making the institutional placement.

There is some beginning experience in dealing with a less advantaged and more minority population in the Veterans Administration hospitals throughout the country. There are now at least 18 hospice or hospice-like programs in the VA that deal with a population that is almost entirely male, frequently minority, frequently without a permanent home and family, and often beset by alcoholism or other social problems. The early experience with these patients is that they require much more time as inpatients, that home care is difficult to provide adequately, and that psychosocial counseling and assistance is much more necessary.[5] It *is* possible to deliver very good hospice care to these patients, but the program organization and philosophy must be considerably different from what is usually considered as hospice in other settings.

Clearly this underrepresentation of certain segments of the population should not be tolerated. Poor and uninsured patients in city or county hospitals need hospice programs as much as middle-class private patients in voluntary hospitals, perhaps even more. Minority patients need hospice programs as much as nonminority patients, perhaps even more. Patients with alcoholism or mental illness or lack of a permanent home and family need hospice programs as much as those not beset by these complications, perhaps even more. Hospices must care for patients across the social and racial spectrum if they are to fulfill their highest ideals and purposes.

Summary

The question "Which patients should hospices serve?" is not so ludicrous as it first seems. It involves consideration of the real role of a hospice, that is, a specialized referral unit for "difficult" deaths versus a general care unit for all deaths. It involves consideration of the basic disease condition that is threatening life, that is, cancer versus other disease causes of death. It involves a review of the socioeconomic and racial compositions of populations being served, in order to ensure that the needs of the *total* community are being met.

Each hospice will answer the question "Which patients should hospices serve?" in a different fashion, but each one should face the question directly and not pretend it doesn't make any difference. Each hospice should review its resources and its potential, should identify which patients it feels it can serve best, and then see to it that these are the ones actually served. An appropriate public policy regarding hospice programs should also identify which patients should be served and which hospices should do the serving; it should then also ensure that the right patients get to the right hospices.

References

1. Saunders, C., Walsh, T. D., and Smith, M. A review of 100 cases of motor neuron disease in a hospice. In: *Hospice: The Living Idea.* Saunders, C., Summers, D. H., and Teller, N., editors. London: Edward Arnold Publishers, 1981.

2. Summers, D. H. The caring team in motor neuron disease. In: *Hospice: The Living Idea.* Saunders, C., Summers, D. H., and Teller, N., editors. London: Edward Arnold Publishers, 1981.

3. Butterfield-Picard, H., and Magno, J. Hospice the adjective, not the noun: The future of a national priority. *American Psychologist.* 1982. 37:1254-59.

4. Care for the terminally ill — an update on hospice issues and operations. Program information letter, U.S. Department of Health and Human Services, Washington, DC, 1981.

5. Krasnow, R., and Wales, J. Palliative Care Program, Wadsworth VA Hospital, Los Angeles. Personal communications, 1982 Nov.

Chapter | 5

Considerations in Hospice Licensure

John D. Blum, J.D., M.S.,
and Dennis A. Robbins, Ph.D., M.P.H.

The development of hospice programs in the United States has been so rapid and so energetic in nature that it has, until recently, outrun any significant consideration of the important issues of licensure and accreditation. In general, emphasis has been mainly on getting programs started and providing service, not on how they would eventually be approved by government agencies or professional organizations.

Within the past few years, as increasingly serious consideration has been given to financing hospice care through public programs or through private health insurance, questions of licensure and accreditation have become much more important and have begun to receive more attention. Several states have passed hospice licensure laws, several organizations have seriously studied the question of hospice accreditation, and the whole question of formal approval of hospice programs has become a much more central concern for everyone interested in hospice programs.

Because the two issues, licensure and accreditation, involve similar questions and are linked in many ways, they are considered in close sequence to each other in this book. However, because they are also significantly different in many of their aspects and because they involve very different types of organizations and structures, they are considered separately. In this chapter, the questions of licensure are reviewed, and the next chapter deals with accreditation.

Differences between Licensure and Accreditation

The terms *licensure* and *accreditation* are frequently used in the same fashion by those unfamiliar with their exact meaning. In fact, they are quite different from one another, and the difference should be known and understood by all who are interested in either the licensing or the accreditation of hospice programs.

Licensure is the granting of a specific privilege by a government authority or agency, permitting acts that would be unlawful in the absence of such permission. Licensure deals with questions of law and statutes and is mandatory for those persons or institutions covered by the licensing requirements.

Accreditation, on the other hand, does not grant specific permission to do anything and certainly does not grant permission to exist or provide services. Instead, it is an organized review of the operation and resources of a program or facility, to determine whether that organization is operating within a certain acceptable level of quality. It compares the operations of that organization against a previously established set of standards or measures of excellence. The accreditation process itself is a voluntary one on the part of the organization being reviewed, and, at least theoretically, the organization could continue to exist and operate without accreditation.

The confusion between licensure and accreditation arises from the frequent use of the *results* of one (for example, accreditation) in the *processes* of the other (for example, licensure). In some situations, the laws may state that licensure will not be granted to unaccredited programs or facilities, making such accreditation a necessary step towards becoming licensed. In the same fashion, the procedures and processes of an accreditation organization may state that accreditation will not be granted to an unlicensed program or facility. The intermingling of the *results* of the individual processes tends to blur the distinction between them.

In the same fashion, both licensure and accreditation may be required for a program or a facility to receive financial reimbursement from a health insurance program, either private or government. By requiring that an organization be both licensed and accredited in order to receive funds, the insurance carrier may inadvertently foster the impression in the mind of the public that the two are the same or that they are necessarily linked in some fashion. It is hoped that the distinction between the two will become clear as the discussion of licensure and accreditation of hospices continues in this chapter and the next.

Rationale for Hospice Licensure

The process of licensing is a complex one that is plagued by numerous difficulties. Nevertheless, there are three primary reasons that make licensure of hospices a necessary process: (1) protection of the public, (2) provision of a legal basis for practice, and (3) assurance of financial reimbursement from third-party payers.

Initially, as is the case with other health care systems, the state has a duty to ensure that an entity within its jurisdiction provides health care in an acceptable fashion. This government responsibility to protect the public prompts the need for an official process to maintain some control over hospice programs. The scope of that control can range from a definition of what can be recognized as a hospice, to a description of which patients such an entity can treat, to a discussion of questions of structure and even tax status.

Clearly the state cannot dictate how health care will be provided on an individual basis, but it can mandate a general treatment format that will affect the individual hospice care process. Very often, the licensure law itself is only the initial stage in the exercise of government control, the actual details of that control being contained in the regulations that are drawn up to fulfill the mandates of the licensing act. The exercise of control over hospices for the purpose of protecting the public emerges most explicitly in the regulations rather than in the licensing law itself; the licensing law may simply make the process of regulation writing possible.

The second reason for hospice licensure is the need to provide hospice organizations with a sound legal basis for operating. Without such a basis in state law, an organization's ability to deliver health care services is highly questionable, and the hospice is vulnerable to potential civil and criminal liability problems. In this sense, licensure represents a fundamental and practical operating consideration that protects the hospice organizations themselves.

It should be pointed out that, at this point, only a few states have specific licensing laws for hospice programs, thus forcing hospices to be licensed under statutes designed for other types of health care programs, such as home health care agencies, nursing homes, special hospitals, and the like. The legal uncertainties created by this form of indirect licensure of hospices are considerable and could create significant problems for hospice programs in the future, particularly the community-based hospice programs that are not part of a larger organization like a hospital or a home health agency. If these community-based hospices cannot be included in a sponsoring hospital or home health agency and if their state does not have a separate hospice licensing law, they may have no real legal existence as a health care program at all. This means that they may not be eligible for accreditation and may not be able to obtain third-party reimbursement for their services.

The final reason for hospice licensure is related to financial reimbursement for hospice programs. Increasingly, the insurance coverage for hospice care is expanding, with both private insurers and the Medicare program now including hospice services as a covered item. In both public and private insurance plans, there is often a requirement that care be given by licensed providers if it is to be eligible for reimbursement.

Difficulties in the Development of Appropriate Hospice Licensing

There are several difficulties related to the development of appropriate hospice licensing that must be noted. The first is the lack of a single, universally accepted organizational model for hospice programs, and the second is the need for licensing legislation that is specific enough to accomplish the necessary regulatory objectives and yet general enough to allow for continued innovation and experimentation in a field that is still young and developing.

With regard to the lack of a universally accepted organizational model for hospice, the wide variation among the hundreds of hospice programs that exist in the United States, both in their form of organization and in the range of services they offer, has already been pointed out in previous chapters. Some hospices are separate and freestanding organizations, whereas others are merely parts of larger parent organizations. Some hospices operate inpatient services of their own, whereas others use the facilities already present in the community. Some hospices offer extensive programs of services that are provided by their own staff, whereas others have very limited staff and prefer to contract for services provided by other organizations. Some hospices rely heavily on unlicensed nonprofessional volunteers to carry out the bulk of the hospice programs' work, whereas others use volunteers in a much more secondary and ancillary capacity.

Although all these programs would probably claim that they adhere to the general standards and principles developed by the National Hospice Organization or by the International Work Group on Death, Dying, and Bereavement, in practice they probably differ significantly in how they implement those standards. Developing a licensing law that would apply equally and fairly to all of them will be an extremely difficult matter.

The second major difficulty related to the development of appropriate hospice licensing legislation is the fact that the hospice movement is still quite young and has considerable growth and development ahead of it. It is important to remember that the first of the modern hospices, St. Christopher's in London, opened its doors only in 1967, and the majority of the currently operating hospices came into existence after 1979. To impose an even loosely structured set of licensing laws on such a new and developing organizational form might well mean the end of the innovation in form and content that has characterized the hospice movement from the beginning.

Tied in with this point is the political reality that licensure laws often reflect the views and values of those encouraging their development. With regard to hospice, this could mean that people with one particular view of hospice (for example, that every hospice program should have its own inpatient beds) might succeed in pushing through legislation that strengthens their particular point of view and possibly weakens others. Future hospice development might then no longer follow the broad and generalized front that it has up to this point but might instead be channeled into a more narrow and particular form that prematurely closes off initiatives that should be encouraged.

State Hospice Licensure and Regulatory Developments

Fifteen states have enacted statutes dealing with hospice. They are: Colorado, Connecticut, Delaware, Florida, Georgia, Illinois, Maryland, Michigan, Montana, New Mexico, New York, Rhode Island, South Carolina, Virginia, and West Virginia. Of this group, the laws of Florida, Illinois, and Virginia are most comprehensive; other states, such as Delaware, Maryland, Michigan, and New York, have hospice bills that are very limited and general, leaving the tasks of providing specificity to state regulators. Legislation in Connecticut dealing with hospice is rather narrow, mentioning hospice in the context of home health agencies (although the hospice regulations in that state are extensive). West Virginia law defines hospice in a bill that sets up a statewide continuum of care board that is mandated to assist local communities in establishing interdisciplinary hospice programs. California's hospice bill merely endorses passage of federal hospice legislation.

Besides legislation, state agencies have developed and promulgated regulations in Colorado, Connecticut, Delaware, Florida, Georgia, Kentucky, Montana, New Mexico, New York, Rhode Island, and Washington to establish specific licensure provisions for hospice programs. In other states, such as Maryland, Michigan, South Carolina, and Virginia, regulations are pending. It is interesting to note that Washington and Kentucky have not passed hospice legislation, and yet fairly detailed regulations have been promulgated in these two states. There is a movement in some states to add hospice regulations to existing regulatory requirements for home health agencies, as was done in Indiana and Texas. Also, some states may consider amending general health facility licensure laws by including hospice, as was done in New Mexico and New Hampshire. A number of states are weighing the possibility of using Joint Commission on Accreditation of Hospitals (JCAH) accreditation standards as the basis for regulation.

In the majority of states where there are not yet specific hospice statutes or regulations, hospices, as previously indicated, are frequently regulated under preexisting categories, often as home health agencies. As entities licensed under other classifications, hospice programs must fulfill special requirements, such as compliance with certificate-of-need legislation that was designed for the initial type of organization being licensed, not for hospices. Hawaii, however, specifically requires by legislation that hospice programs comply with the state certificate-of-need requirements, in their own right, regardless of the category under which they may be licensed.[1]

The task of drafting hospice legislation or regulations is greatly complicated by the fact that consensus has not been reached about the essential elements of what any hospice program, regardless of the model utilized, must provide. The lack of agreement about what the essential characteristics of hospice are can be seen by examining hospice definitions that have been adopted in state laws and regulations. For the most part, states that have defined hospice have done so in general terms, with the exception of hospice definitions that refer only to one model, such as the state of Washington definition of hospice care center facilities. In reviewing existing state definitions, one finds that they tend to be a delineation of general services that must be provided in coordinated programs of care; such definitions do not address the issue of identifying the essence of what any hospice program must be.

A recent representative example of a hospice definition can be found in West Virginia law. Hospice is defined as

> (2) a coordinated program of home and inpatient care provided directly or through an agreement under the direction of an identifiable hospice administration which provides palliative and supportive medical and other health services to terminally ill patients and their families. Hospice utilizes a medically directed interdisciplinary team. A hospice program of care provides care to meet the physical, psychological, social, spiritual and other special needs which are experienced during the final stages of illness, and during dying and bereavement.[2]

The key elements present in this definition include coordinated program, home and inpatient care, identifiable administration, palliative and supportive health and medical services, terminally ill patients and their families, interdisciplinary teams, and addressing a range of needs during the final stages of illness and dying and during bereavement. These elements are for the most part found in most hospice definitions.

Perhaps the most general definition of hospice is that adopted by the state of Michigan. The Michigan definition reads:

> (4) "Hospice" means a health care program which provides a coordinated set of services rendered at home or in outpatient or institutional settings for individuals suffering from a disease or condition with a terminal prognosis.[3]

Such a definition clearly provides great flexibility to state regulators to develop specific regulations that can accommodate a variety of hospice models.

In contrast to the Michigan definition and to a lesser extent that of West Virginia is the definition of hospice incorporated into Florida law. The Florida definition states:

> (2) "Hospice" means an autonomous, centrally administered, non-profit, as defined in chapter 617, medically directed, nurse-coordinated program providing a continuum of home, outpatient, and homelike inpatient care for the terminally ill patient and his family. It employs an interdisciplinary team to assist in providing palliative and supportive care to meet the special needs arising out of the physical, emotional, spiritual, social, and economic stresses which are experienced during the final stages of illness and during dying and bereavement. This care is available 24 hours a day, 7 days a week, and is provided on the basis of need regardless of inability to pay.[4]

Florida's approach to hospice definition represents a stronger conviction of how a hospice must be structured than was evident in the definition of either West Virginia or Michigan. Inclusion of specific requirements, such as those mandating that hospice be a nurse-coordinated program with an ongoing broad continuum of services and excluding for-profit operations, represents both a conviction of the nature of hospice programs, and a strong bias that special safeguards are needed to prevent potential abuses.

Perhaps the most detailed definition of hospice comes from the regulations of Washington State.[5] Washington's definition covers only hospice care centers that are either freestanding or separately licensed sections or areas of another licensed facility. As a definition that is facility-oriented, the Washington regulation tends to focus more on the structural nature of a hospice than on the essence of the concept.

The initial efforts of state regulators in attempting to define hospice should not be viewed with undue criticism, for the difficulty in this area reflects uncertainties in the field at large. The definitional challenge is indicative of the problems of drafting effective regulations in an evolving area. The uncertainty in characterizing the nature of the hospice concept should not be used as a reason for states to abandon regulation; instead, the uncertainty ought to act as an incentive for them to regulate. In fact, states having a duty to safeguard public health and safety in this area should strive to clarify the elements of hospice in their jurisdiction.

As mentioned previously, the majority of states at present regulate hospice programs within the framework of existing licensure classifications. In the various states, hospices are regulated as special hospitals, skilled nursing facilities, home health agencies, or other special organizations, depending on the types of hospices that exist in those states and on the forms of licensure already in force. Many states have not felt a need to license or regulate hospice programs yet because of the limited number of programs and patients involved and the early stage of development of the field. Some states chose not to develop specific hospice regulations because of the belief that hospice was too new a concept and should be allowed to develop prior to creating new regulatory controls. In other states, great uncertainty existed about what hospices were and how they functioned, with a resulting lack of consensus about what type of legislation was needed. In a few other states, proponents of one outlook or another sponsored legislation that supported their specific view of hospice, and that was the legislation that eventually passed.

The current posture of states toward hospice regulation must be viewed in relation to the certification requirements for participating in the Medicare hospice benefits. Although significant attention has been focused on the reimbursement aspects of Medicare coverage, perhaps equally important to the structure of hospice organization are the conditions for participation in the Medicare benefits. These conditions of participation are not licensing statutes at all; nevertheless, they mandate certain forms of organization and services that hospices must follow if they wish to be reimbursed by Medicare. As a result, practically they are just as important as the state licensing laws that exist.

It is unclear what the position of the individual states will be with regard to hospice licensure and regulation. One school of thought argues that states should not take independent regulatory action until some experience with the federal regulations is established. In this way, state efforts that are eventually developed could be better coordinated with the Medicare requirements for participation.

The Medicare regulations do not exclude state regulatory involvement, however, and another school of thought suggests that they actually encourage state legislators to become active in this area. In those states where such laws exist, the federal regulations require that state hospice licensure laws must be adhered to, prior to Medicare certification. In this way, although the federal Medicare program has assumed increased influence over the hospice movement because of Medicare's great financial power, each state can retain control of hospice development within the state by the establishment of specific licensing laws.

It is unclear at this point how much flexibility states will ultimately possess in sanctioning alternatives that differ from Medicare criteria. A fair degree of discretion may be exercised by states, and the perceived need to exercise that discretionary power can be viewed as a primary incentive for state hospice licensure and/or regulation.

Existing State Licensure Laws for Hospices

The Florida statute enacted in 1978 and amended in 1981 and 1982 is now the most detailed hospice licensure law in the country.[6] The Florida law specifies the kinds of services a hospice must provide, as well as requirements for staffing, record keeping and confidentiality, yearly licensing, and certificate of need. Admission to a Florida hospice may be authorized only by a physician and requires the express request and informed consent of both patient and family. It is interesting to note that the Florida statute does not limit hospice care to terminally ill patients whose prognosis for life is less than one year but views this care as appropriate for anyone suffering from illness for which a cure is no longer possible. A recent amendment to the Florida statute requested that detailed regulatory guidelines dealing with all aspects of hospice operations be developed, and these regulations have recently been promulgated.

The Virginia statute is less detailed than Florida's, yet in the small field of hospice legislation, it stands out as one of the most comprehensive licensure laws.[7] The Virginia law defines a hospice broadly as a coordinated program of home and inpatient care; the statute specifies that to be eligible for hospice, patients have life expectancies of six months or less. Besides providing definitions of key elements (such as hospice, patient, family, administration, and interdisciplinary team), the Virginia law establishes a system of licensure for hospice programs controlled by the state commissioner of health. Licensure is to be activated by development and adoption of a series of regulations dealing with, at minimum, personnel, coordination of services, management, operations, record keeping, and utilization review. The statute requires that the Virginia Department of Health regulators coordinate the application of hospice regulations so that facilities already licensed (such as home health agencies) are not mandated to meet duplicative requirements. The commissioner of health in the licensing process has the authority to conduct periodic examinations of licensed hospices. All hospices are required to renew their licenses annually, and the only hospice programs exempt from the licensure requirement are those run by a religious organization providing just spiritual counseling with no drug or medical intervention.

Other state legislation that provides for hospice licensure can be found in Michigan and Maryland. The Michigan law requires that all hospice programs be licensed by the state's health department.[8] The law places total program responsibility on the owners, operators, or governing body of the hospice. Services are to be coordinated so that a hospice patient can be transferred from one setting to another with minimal disruption and discontinuity of care. The Michigan statute further requires use of interdisciplinary teams and outlines specific admission requirements. For the most part, the delineation of specific requirements for licensure and operation are not present in the Michigan law but are left to the state's department of health to develop through the rule-making process.

Under Maryland law, hospice is defined as a facility, separate from any other facility, that offers a hospice care program, namely, "a coordinated interdisciplinary program for meeting the special physical, psychological, spiritual and social needs of dying individuals and their families."[9] Maryland requires that all hospices be licensed by the state Secretary of Health and that prior to licensure, a certificate of need be obtained. Unlike other statutes, the term of licensure is three years. The Maryland statute does not delineate specific operational requirements but, rather, authorizes the Secretary of Health, in consultation with the Maryland Hospice Reimbursement Study Commission, to develop rules and regulations for medical personnel, dietary, nursing, pastoral care, pharmaceutical, and social worker services. It is interesting to note that Maryland, by 1982 statute, requires that individual, group, and not-for-profit health service plans providing health coverage in the state offer hospice care services to their insureds.[10]

Existing State Hospice Regulations

Although it is helpful to examine state enabling legislation, state regulations that have been developed either pursuant to a statute or independent of one offer considerable guidance on how state government can shape the structure and dictate the operation of hospice programs. Of promulgated state hospice regulations, Florida's stand out as being the most comprehensive. The Florida regulations cover the following areas: statement of purpose, definitions, licensure required, licensure procedure, governing body and management, medical direction, coordinated care program, dietary services, pharmaceutical services, diagnostic services, clergy and/or counseling services, social services, volunteer services, infection control, interdisciplinary care records, outpatient services, bereavement services, housekeeping services, and physical plant requirements. In each of the areas mentioned, the Florida regulations are quite detailed and should be examined as valuable reference points. For purposes of this chapter, only two sections will be explored, the coordinated care program and bereavement services.[11]

In the coordinated care program, Florida regulations require that the overall program of patient-family care be coordinated by a registered nurse who has at least three years of supervisory experience. The nurse (termed the *patient-family care coordinator*) is responsible for creating and monitoring a hospice staffing for inpatient, outpatient, and home care. Nursing ratios specified in an eight-hour shift include at least one registered nurse to ten patients, one licensed nurse to five patients, and one patient care staff person to three patients. Other duties of the patient-family care coordinator include creating a plan for decision making among representative disciplines on the interdisciplinary care team and developing and implementing a plan to assist the nursing staff in meeting collective and individual responsibilities specified in each patient-family interdisciplinary plan of care.

Under the coordinated care program section, each hospice is required to establish a joint practice committee that is responsible for providing ongoing evaluation and review of hospice services and patient-family care. The committee is to be composed of a hospice physician, a registered nurse, a social worker, a member of the clergy or a counselor, a hospice volunteer, the patient or family member currently cared for, an outside physician, and an outside member of the clergy plus a pharmacist, a dietitian, a housekeeper, a medical records practitioner, a physical or occupational therapist, and a speech pathologist.

In this section, the unit of care is defined as including patient and family; *family* is used very broadly to include not only legally related individuals but anyone whom the patient considers to be family. The care is to be provided by the hospice interdisciplinary team, which, at the minimum, consists of a physician, a registered nurse, a social worker, a member of the clergy or a counselor, and a volunteer. On admission to a hospice, the patient-family is to be assigned to an interdisciplinary team, which is to have primary responsibility to the patient-family through all components of the hospice program. (On occasion, however, more than one hospice team may be providing care to one patient and family.)

The interdisciplinary team is responsible for drafting a care plan based on an assessment of the physical, psychosocial, and spiritual needs of the patient and the coping ability of the patient and the family. The plan must include specific goals, the services to be rendered, and (when they are indicated) a drug therapy and bereavement plan. The plan must include skilled palliative care for the patient, the goal of which is to control physical pain; skilled psychological and spiritual counseling for the patient and family; and bereavement counseling for the family.

Besides developing, documenting, and monitoring a patient-family's plan of care, the interdisciplinary team is required to provide a constant communication link with the family, document all requests for hospice care, and ensure provision of services 24 hours a day, 7 days a week. The team is required to offer continuity of services for the patient-family regardless of the setting, and finally, if possible, the interdisciplinary team is to remain constant from admission to the hospice through the bereavement period.

The Florida hospice regulation section covering bereavement services requires provision of such services to families both before and after the patient's death; these services are to extend one year beyond the death of the patient. The goal of bereavement services is to offer counseling to assist families in understanding and coping with their grief and in maintaining their normal lives as much as possible. Bereavement services must be consistent with the interdisciplinary patient-family care plan, and their provision needs to be carefully documented. Insofar as possible, bereavement counseling is to be coordinated with the family's cleric, as well as with available community resources.

Connecticut, Delaware, and New York have developed detailed hospice regulations, and such regulations are now pending in other states. The Connecticut regulations, prompted by the pathfinding experience of the New Haven hospice group, were the first state regulations promulgated in the country. Although portions of the Connecticut regulations apply to both kinds of inpatient hospice program, they are clearly tailored toward the freestanding hospice facility. The Connecticut regulations, in fact, are contained within the framework of that state's short-term hospital regulations.[12]

The New York regulations were developed in 1979 to establish specific requirements for the creation and administration of hospice projects.[13] These regulations lay down basic definitions, hospice application procedures, and a detailed section concerning hospice organization and administration. Within the organization and administration section, requirements for hospice governance, administration, staffing, patient referral and admissions, patient-family care services, records or reports, and patient or program evaluation are detailed. As of this writing, New York is in the process of updating its hospice regulatory program.

In Kentucky and Washington, state agencies have developed regulations for hospice institutions; neither state has any special hospice legislation. The Kentucky regulations mandate that the state health facilities and health services certificate-of-need and licensure board license all hospice programs operating within the state whether the hospice is freestanding or operated by another licensed provider.[14] Kentucky licensure requires that programs establish policies dealing with acceptance of patients, interdisciplinary plans of care, quality care audits, personnel policies and procedures, and use of volunteers. In addition, the regulations include other general administrative and/or organizational requirements such as medical record policies, personnel requirements, and handling of contractual arrangements. Each hospice is required, at the minimum, to have a medical director, an administrator, and a registered nurse patient-care coordinator. Although hospices in Kentucky have considerable leeway in contracting out for services, certain services must be provided directly. These include coordination of medical aspects of a hospice program; patient-family assessment of physical, psychological, spiritual, social, and economic needs; development and coordination of a plan of care; patient counseling; family bereavement counseling; and education and training of staff, volunteers, and family members.

Washington State hospice regulations promulgated by the state board of health require licensure for freestanding hospice care centers. The regulations read: "The purpose...is to provide minimal standards for safety and adequate care of terminally ill individuals who choose to receive palliative rather than curative care and treatment for varying periods of time in a segregated, organized, specialized hospital or health care center." What was developed by the Washington board of health is a set of regulations that provides very comprehensive requirements for hospice facilities, including definitions, licensure requirements, and specifications for governance, staffing, patient care services, food and dietary services, infection control, pharmaceutical service, clinical records, and physical environment and equipment.[15]

Some provisions of the Washington regulations are very specific. For example, in the area of food and dietary services, the Washington regulation is broken into eight parts, requiring management of the program by an individual trained in food service, use of nutritional and dietary consultation, and nutritionally balanced meals with consideration given to patients' ethnic preferences. Therapeutic diets are to be recommended by physicians, with the assistance of a therapeutic diet manual approved by both a dietitian and the hospice medical director. Other food and diet requirements concern storage, refrigeration, dining areas, food service sanitation and development, and use of written policies and procedures for matters dealing with food preparation, storage, and cleaning.

The state of Alabama, through its department of public health, has issued a set of regulatory guidelines for hospice programs that are very comprehensive, although not yet binding. The Alabama hospice guidelines were drafted as supplements to state nursing home and hospital regulations and as such are very much facility-oriented. The guidelines were based on requirements of the National Hospice Organization and Medicare/Medicaid skilled nursing facility regulations. The 29 pages of Alabama guidelines include sections on definitions; governance; infection control; medical records; medical staff; nursing, pharmaceutical, dietary, pastoral care, volunteer, and outpatient services; hospice-based home care; and physical facility requirements.

Public Law 97-248

No review of state regulatory activity would be complete without some reference to federal activity in the area, because the federal regulatory activity will have a direct influence on future developments in the states. Although it is not the intent here to analyze P.L. 97-248 in detail, some brief observations are in order.[16]

The federal statute defines hospice programs in terms of items and services that must be offered but does not attempt to define the hospice concept itself.[17] A hospice program in the federal statute is to be a public or private organization that offers 24-hour services to terminally ill patients (those with less than six months to live) in the home, on an outpatient basis, and on a short-term inpatient basis. The statute lists a number of services and items hospices must provide for Medicare, including nursing care, physical and/or occupational therapy, medical social services, home health aid, medical supplies, physician services, short-term inpatient care, and counseling. In this list, nursing care, physician-directed medical social services, physician services, and counseling must be provided directly. Other details included in the federal statute are very similar to existing state law requirements, such as use of an interdisciplinary care team, creation of individual plans of care, and the use of volunteers. Major portions of the federal law concern reimbursement policy for hospice and mandate the development of regulatory measures and special studies. It is interesting to note that the federal statute prohibits reimbursement for either counseling or bereavement services.

Also, under the regulations a hospice patient (one who is diagnosed as being terminally ill with six months or less to live) must personally elect the hospice benefit, which lasts for three periods totalling 210 days. By so electing, a patient generally waives his or her rights to receive benefits under other parts of Medicare. The entire hospice benefit is subject to a cap of $6,500 per patient, and each certified program is required to provide the bulk of its services on an outpatient or home care basis.

Discussion and Considerations for the Future

After a review of all the diverse state licensing and regulatory actions regarding hospice programs,[18] what general observations can be made and what general lessons can be learned? Going further, what considerations should be kept in mind when approaching hospice licensure and regulation in the future? Several general observations can be made about the present situation with regard to licensing and regulation of hospices by the individual states.

First, it is clear after reviewing the various state statutes and regulations that there is no one universally accepted model in place at the present time. There is great variation in the form and content of the statutes, in the agencies assigned to implement them, and even in the apparent purpose and intent of the laws themselves. Certain licensing laws focus much more vigorously on the freestanding hospice model and consequently assign considerable emphasis to physical and structural considerations rather than program content. Other laws and regulations seem to have community-based home care programs in mind and, therefore, focus their attention more on services that must be offered by a hospice program and less on physical or structural considerations.

Second, there is considerable unease among leaders in the hospice field about more specific hospice licensure and regulatory control at this time. Some have reservations because they believe that premature licensing could have a potentially negative impact on the continued innovation and development of hospice programs. Even for those hospice experts who do believe that some form of licensure and regulatory activity is needed, there is no agreement on what form that licensure should take and what content the regulatory activity should have. There are individual hospice leaders with strong opinions one way or the other, but there is no industrywide consensus at this time.

Third, there also seems to be a hesitancy on the part of state authorities and hospice experts to advocate any vigorous approach to state licensing and regulation of hospice programs until the federal Medicare regulations and conditions of participation are well understood and completely tested in practice. Although it might be argued that now would be the time for an aggressive approach by a state government that wanted to control the development of hospice programs in its state, there seems to be no rush to fill this void. It seems apparent that the federal Medicare regulations and conditions of participation will shape the individual state actions in this area rather than the other way around.

Given the various uncertainties and differences that exist in the present licensing and regulation of hospice programs, what considerations should be kept in mind when approaching the subject in the future? What general guidelines can be laid down to help in the development of these activities in the years to come?

First, although there is a growing need to have appropriate licensing and regulatory machinery in place, states should probably approach the development of this machinery with caution, because the hospice movement is still in its formative stages. Premature or poorly drawn licensing laws or regulatory controls could do considerable harm to what is still a developing field. There is probably no great hurry to have a full, completely detailed licensing and regulatory effort in place, and states should probably begin the developmental process now, with the view that further, more exact modifications will be made as practical experience with hospice grows.

Second, states should be clear in their purpose for engaging in hospice licensure or regulation, so that the ensuing statutes will actually serve that purpose well. States should not proceed until there is a broad general consensus throughout the state as to what a hospice is and what it is supposed to do. States should specifically avoid allowing the licensure or regulatory process to be captured by one opinion group or another, thereby isolating or excluding other significant opinions and groups.

Third, there should be a general recognition that hospice is defined as a program of service that can be delivered by a number of organizational models. This means that any attempt at licensure or regulation of hospices must deal with both aspects of hospice—the service content of the program, and the various possible vehicles for delivering these services to people. State licensing laws or regulations regarding hospice should not confuse the "medium" (that is, the *means* of delivering hospice services) with the "message" (that is, the *content* of those services themselves). Licensure laws should probably deal with the means of delivering hospice service to people, whereas regulations should probably deal with the content of those services.

In the event that states do pass hospice licensing statutes, grandfather clauses should probably be provided for already established programs so that they can continue to function without disruption of their services. As an alternative, it may be necessary to establish a time limit within which existing hospice programs can comply with newly developed licensing requirements. It would be extremely unfortunate if new licensing or regulatory requirements forced the closure of programs that had begun in good faith and that had led the way in development of the hospice idea, but that for some reason may not meet a set of newly developed criteria or standards.

In view of the possible difficulty in developing hospice licensure laws and regulatory controls, states should consider other more flexible means of control. One alternative is the use of operating protocols. The hospice program itself might be allowed to develop a protocol outlining the details of its operation, its services, staffing, management, finances, and the like. This operating protocol might be developed with some general guidance from a state department of health and would have the dual advantage of allowing the state to exert sufficient control (that is, by approval or disapproval of the operating protocol), while at the same time providing the flexibility necessary to support and encourage new programs in a still-developing field.

Finally, as a general consideration, it will be important for those involved in the licensure and regulation of hospices to regularly reevaluate and reappraise whatever approach has been taken in a particular area. The next few years will be critical because a series of patterns will probably be set for hospice licensure and regulation; these procedures must be continuously reviewed so that necessary changes can be made before the pattern is established permanently. Five years from now, today's preliminary attempts at licensure and regulation may well be viewed as permanent, and alterations then may be difficult to carry out. Continuous reevaluation and modification of these processes will ensure that the permanent statutes that eventually emerge will be the best possible.

References

1. Hawaii Revised Statutes Sec. 323D-41(7).
2. West Virginia, H.B. 1921 Sec. 16-5D-2.
3. Michigan Civil Law Sec. 333.21404.
4. Florida Public Health Sec. 460.601.
5. Washington Annotated Code 248-21-002.

6. Florida Statutes Annotated Sec. 400.601-400.615.

7. Code of Virginia, Chapter 5, Title 32.162.1-162-6.

8. Michigan Civil Law Sec. 333.21401-21421.

9. Annotated Maryland Code, 19-901-19-913.

10. Annotated Maryland Code, Art. 48A Sec. 477W; Art. 48A Sec. 470Q; Art. 48A, Sec. 361E.

11. Florida Department of Health and Rehabilitation Services, 10D-80.07, 10D-80.20.

12. Regulations of the Connecticut Department of Health, Sec. 19-13-D46, Jan. 1979.

13. New York State Regulations, Public Health Sec. 2801 (1,10).

14. 902 Kentucky A.R. 20:140, Operations and Services, Hospice.

15. Washington Annotated Code 248-21.

16. The Tax Equity and Fiscal Responsibility Act of 1982, Sec. 122. Public Law 97-248, Congress of the United States.

17. Guidelines Supplement to the Rules, Regulations, and Standards for Nursing Homes (301.2 Skilled Nursing Home) and Hospitals (301.2 Combination Classification) with Hospice Services. Washington, DC: Department of Health and Human Services, Health Care Financing Administration, 1983.

18. At time of publication, hospice regulatory activity was pending in the following states: California, Indiana, Iowa, Massachusetts, New York, North Carolina, Ohio, Oregon, South Carolina, Vermont, and Wisconsin.

Chapter 6

Considerations in Hospice Accreditation

Claire Tehan, M.A.

Within the past few years, an expanding interest in a formal accreditation process for hospice programs has been spurred by the prospect of reimbursement for hospice care by Medicare and the need to identify acceptable hospice programs. Much of the interest, however, long predates any consideration of Medicare reimbursement; rather, it arose from the genuine desire of early hospice leaders to ensure that all hospice programs met a high standard of excellence. Even before formation of the National Hospice Organization (NHO), groups of prominent hospice leaders were meeting and drawing up minimal acceptable standards of care for hospices.[1,2] Later, when the NHO came into existence, these early efforts were incorporated into the NHO statement *Standards of a Hospice Program of Care,* which appeared first in 1979 and then in a revised form in 1981.[3,4]

Licensure, Certification, Accreditation, and Deemed Status

As mentioned in the previous chapter, licensure, certification, and accreditation are frequently confused with one another; thus, it is necessary to clarify these terms.

Licensure is an attempt by the state to define and enforce minimum requirements of operation. Licensure has evolved as a means of protecting the public through the application of legal restrictions and controls. Only a few states have enacted hospice licensure laws; many hospice programs function within, and are reimbursed under, existing licensure categories such as home health agencies, acute hospitals, or skilled nursing facilities. Those hospice programs that exist in states with no specific licensure laws and that do not otherwise qualify under existing licensure categories for hospitals, home health agencies, or nursing homes actually operate in a legal vacuum. Unable to obtain licensure on their own and unqualified to obtain licensure in an existing category, these hospice programs operate without defined minimum standards. Community-based, volunteer-organized hospice programs (which represent a significant portion of programs in the United States) fall into this category and face an uncertain legal future.

Certification is a process by which programs or facilities are reviewed to determine whether they meet minimum requirements for providing services to the beneficiaries of government third-party payers, primarily Medicare and Medicaid. The federal Medicare program, for example, maintains a set of conditions for health care providers who want to participate in the Medicare program. If a hospital or nursing home wishes to care for Medicare patients and receive reimbursement, it must be certified by Medicare as having satisfactorily met these conditions.

Accreditation is a voluntary process in which a health care facility or program chooses to be measured against a set of professional standards for that type of program. These standards are generally established by the field itself or in cooperation with leading members of that field. It reflects a commitment to continuous evaluation of the quality of work and an ongoing effort to improve quality. It does not have the force of law, but frequently legislative, regulatory, or reimbursement bodies refer to accreditation standards in the course of their efforts. Such reference has led to some confusion about the nature of accreditation.

The designation of *deemed status* for the Medicare program is a good example of crossover and possible confusion of the voluntary accreditation process and the quasi-regulatory effects of voluntary accreditation.

Accreditation in the health care industry is not mandated, but passage of the 1965 Medicare-Medicaid legislation made having accredited status a distinct benefit for an organization. The 1965 Social Security Amendments provided that hospitals accredited by the Joint Commmission on Accreditation of Hospitals (JCAH) were deemed to be in compliance with most of the Medicare conditions of participation for hospital providers. This made it unnecessary for JCAH-accredited hospitals to undergo separate federal certification inspection in order to participate in the Medicare program and receive reimbursement for the care of Medicare patients. Hospitals that were not accredited by JCAH, on the other hand, could only participate in the Medicare and Medicaid programs after passing a federally funded, state-conducted certification survey.

With respect to hospice reimbursement, a hospice program must be certified by Medicare as meeting the conditions of participation before it becomes eligible to receive Medicare funds. This certification can be given by a national accrediting body such as the Joint Commission on Accreditation of Hospitals, but Medicare, if it wishes, can also contract with and arrange for state government certification in each of the 50 states. The major problem that arises from multiple state certification efforts, however, is that of equivalency — of being sure that all the individual certification efforts in the different states are carried out in the same fashion, using the same standards. The presence of a single national accreditation organization obviously avoids that difficulty.

A slightly different problem arises when a state handling certification also has a licensing law, and the state government is responsible for both licensing and certification. In this case, the two procedures might have different purposes and therefore might use two different sets of standards, each of which is appropriate for one purpose but possibly not for the other.

Value of the Accreditation Process

One obvious benefit of accreditation arises from its external use by those outside the field who make judgments about the quality or excellence of one program or another. Perhaps an even greater value of accreditation arises from its internal use within the field to stimulate a designated standard of excellence. The real significance of accreditation is its power to stimulate, organize, and give objectivity to the kind of self-evaluation and planning that is essential to improved quality.

Accreditation proponents believe the system can foster excellence in a field as much by the collective process of developing and maintaining an accreditation process, as by the efforts of individual workers or programs who attain accreditation for themselves or their programs. The decision to establish an accreditation process sets into motion a number of positive forces within a particular field.

The first step toward accreditation involves the workers in a particular field who come together and develop objectives and agree on standards of excellence for their work. This effort forces the workers to confront their work directly, to understand it as completely as possible, and to specify their beliefs and standards in writing. This important first step reflects the maturation of a field of work or a system of care, a step that frequently goes unrecognized.

The next step in an accreditation process is the development of specific criteria that measure whether a particular standard of excellence has been attained. This forces a profession or field to move from general standards and statements of values to a more specific, measurable outline of definite things that must be done or events that must take place. The development of criteria forces those in a field to be increasingly more specific and more knowledgeable about the details of their work.

Usually, when an accreditation process is considered, it calls for the support of the entire field; at the very least, the support of the leadership is essential. The need for this consensus pushes members of the field or their leaders to come together and to assert in a tangible way that excellence in their field is important — important enough to warrant the expenditure of valuable time and energy on the process of accreditation.

Once the accreditation process is established, the cornerstone of the process usually is some form of self-study or self-evaluation that is required of all programs seeking accreditation. This is generally a major enterprise and requires considerable time and commitment from an organization, not only to complete the self-study process, but to continuously address problems identified in the self-study. This includes extensive review of the program's policies and practices, attempts to compare organizational performance in certain objective areas against previously established standards, and an exhaustive review of the organization's mission, goals, and operations.

When a profession or field decides to establish an accreditation process, it simultaneously commits itself to providing consultation to member programs as they strive to meet the standards. In this way, efforts to improve the program are assisted as the organization pursues its quest to achieve accreditation. At the same time, the profession or field has a means for continuously shaping the values and influencing the performance of those being accredited. An accreditation process is really the explicit statement of a field's intrinsic values, and its existence makes possible a continuous review and affirmation of those values.

The accreditation process is not without its critics. In an era of antiregulatory sentiment, there has been considerable feeling about much of the tedious, detailed inspection related to accreditation. Some critics suggest that although accreditation may appear voluntary, health care has become so credential- and accreditation-conscious that it is really mandatory, not voluntary. In addition, it has been argued that utilizing the norms of established institutions and programs in an accreditation process tends to discourage innovation and experimentation. This perspective has obvious implications for innovative hospice programs that are still experimental in nature and have considerable development ahead of them.

Others have suggested that an accreditation process developed by representatives from the field being accredited actually makes the process a self-serving one, from which the public is excluded and in which the public interest is not well served. Another complaint is that required paperwork, documentation, and detailed preparation for inspection draw attention away from delivering good care and induce a slavish attention to correctly completed forms and documents. A final perspective on accreditation suggests that the process is too closely tied with state and federal bureaucracies and has lost its freshness and vigor. The result, according to this viewpoint, is a rather dulled legal or regulatory process.

Need for Accreditation

The need for a national hospice accreditation process seems apparent to most thoughtful observers of the hospice field. The United States hospice movement began in the mid-1970s with the opening of the Connecticut hospice; by 1983 there were approximately 1,200 hospice programs in existence or preparing to open their doors. This startling growth has occurred in the past three years and has been characterized by the development of a wide variety of models, carried out in a variety of settings under diverse sponsorship. In the face of this phenomenal growth, the need for some standardization and uniformity around an accepted standard of excellence becomes overwhelming. The November 1983 inclusion of hospice care within the scope of Medicare benefits will undoubtedly result in an explosion of new hospice programs throughout the country and a correspondingly greater need for evaluation and review of all programs.

In addition, many hospice providers fear that the new programs will take improper advantage of the Medicare reimbursement simply because they do not have the long history of commitment to hospice care that the existing programs have. In fact, there will be many reasons for new hospice programs. They may increase when it is felt there is a need or because an enthusiastic group of volunteers is interested in making it work. Others will simply develop because it is good business, because of additional revenue, or because it is a popular service that every complete, competitive hospital should have. An accreditation program would, at a minimum, ensure that the field has some control over the inherent values and the actual form of the programs that develop. At the same time, accreditation procedures ensure that the new programs will be scrutinized and reviewed in light of the perspective and experience of those who have advanced the field to what it is today.

Most important, accreditation will assure both the public and the payers of care that this rapidly developing field is policing itself and that an accepted standard of excellence is being achieved by all accredited programs. The great enthusiasm for hospice care among the providers and the patients and families being cared for is clear. Yet, there is considerable uncertainty among some licensing agencies, insurance companies, hospital executives, and legislators about the next phase of development in the hospice movement. The credibility of a strong accreditation program would ease the concerns of these important constituencies.

Major Concerns regarding Hospice Accreditation

Currently, a number of concerns are being expressed within the hospice movement concerning the subject of accreditation. As accreditation draws closer, it is obvious that new issues will move into the limelight.

Many hospice workers see accreditation as a standardized, bureaucratic process that threatens the creativity and ingenuity of programs it is meant to improve. Most hospice programs reflect the particular philosophy of their founders and the specific circumstances in the community served. Many feel that the development of national standards and the exercise of national oversight authority irreparably damage the local program's sense of initiative, pertinence, and control.

An additional concern about the accrediting process is cost. Most hospices evolved in a setting of minimal to nonexistent financial support. Against this backdrop, the cost of an accreditation survey may be prohibitively expensive. An initial JCAH survey found that most hospice programs could allocate up to $1,000 for accreditation, but many expressed serious doubts about accreditation if the costs were higher. Because the actual costs of accreditation could be much more than $1,000, there is consternation, particularly in the smaller programs, about the inability to afford ongoing accreditation.

There is a very real fear that the required amount and degree of specificity of data and documentation in an accreditation could be excessive. Most hospice programs have very simple organizational structures with limited administrative and clerical staff. Their capacity to produce the documentation required may not be very great. If they do produce what is required, there is apprehension that it will be at the expense of removing personnel from important patient care activities to take care of paperwork.

Another frequently discussed question is whether the field is ready for accreditation at this time. Many hospice programs are still evolving and emerging, and it may not yet be possible to capture the essence of all the diverse forms of hospice care in a single accreditation format, no matter how well intentioned. These critics believe that premature accreditation would result in two negative outcomes: (1) accreditation would not be sensitive to local variations and thus would be unable to adequately evaluate and support what a particular program was actually doing; and (2) a hospice program that did not fit a particular model would be required to do things that were inappropriate for that program.

Indeed, many critics of hospice accreditation express the concern that one group or segment of the hospice movement could gain control of the accreditation process and use it to promote a particular model or form of hospice at the expense of others. Just as with licensing, the accreditation process will possess significant power to affect the values and internal organization of hospice programs, and if used to foster one form of care over another, the ultimate result of accreditation might be an unintentional crippling or constraining of the field.

The final and probably most important criticism of accreditation is that it may not work because there sometimes appears to be no relationship between accredited status and the actual quality of care delivered. There are instances in other fields in which individual programs or facilities have received accredited status but have not delivered good care. The reality is that this situation is the result of an inadequate accrediting process that is not well designed or vigorously implemented, rather than the fault of accreditation itself. In addition, the creation of an accreditation process will not accomplish anything by itself; it must also be used properly.

Selection of an Accrediting Body

As mentioned earlier, leaders in the hospice movement have been developing standards for hospice care since the early 1970s. Paralleling this interest has been an ongoing internal dialogue within the National Hospice Organization about who should implement or enforce those standards, whether through accreditation or some other process. Some leaders thought that NHO should take on the task of establishing standards and evaluating its own members, but others felt that it might be better for the public and patients, as well as for hospice and NHO itself, if some neutral, external accrediting body assumed that responsibility.

In the early 1980s, NHO began preliminary discussions with a number of existing organizations that seemed to be potential accreditors for hospice programs. Included in these discussions were the Joint Commission on Accreditation of Hospitals, the National League for Nursing, the American Public Health Association, the National Association of Home Health Agencies, the California Medical Association, and the Accreditation Association for Ambulatory Health Care.

Rather quickly JCAH was acknowledged as the most prominent and experienced accrediting agency operating in the health care field. Further, the organization had the advantage of active participation with the Medicare programs and extensive familiarity with Medicare requirements and operations. It also, however, had a history of being very actively involved with hospitals and was perceived by some hospice leaders as possibly too hospital-oriented for a program of care initially begun in reaction to unsatisfactory hospital care for the dying.

In 1981, NHO considered the merits of creating its own accreditation program and decided that obvious conflict-of-interest allegations would eventually defeat a self-regulating process. In addition, the high costs of developing an accreditation process that NHO could not afford provided further merit for rejecting the idea. Finally, it was felt that an NHO process would result in unnecessary duplication of effort in light of the JCAH process.

NHO made the decision in 1981 to work with JCAH to explore the possibility of developing an accreditation program for hospices. JCAH applied for and received a two-year grant from the Kellogg Foundation to study the feasibility of hospice accreditation. An advisory committee was established that included representatives from NHO, the American Medical Association, the National League for Nursing, the American Psychiatric Association, the American Hospital Association, the National Conference of Christians and Jews, the American Psychological Association, the National Association of Social Workers, the Health Insurance Association of America, the national Blue Cross and Blue Shield associations, the Health Standards and Quality Bureau of the U.S. Department of Health and Human Services, and the Association of Community Cancer Centers. A small staff was hired and preliminary studies were begun to determine what hospice programs felt about accreditation and to learn more about what JCAH's role might be.

As part of the project, a major effort was made to identify all existing hospices as well as those that were being formed. More than 800 hospice programs in various stages of development were identified, and a hospice survey questionnaire was mailed to them. The questionnaire was designed to elicit information about the programs themselves and to investigate the need and desire for accreditation.

About 77 percent of the programs responded, and a number of significant findings related to accreditation were reported.[5] Substantially all of the programs (81 percent) felt a need for voluntary accreditation, and even more (92 percent) said they would participate if an accreditation program was developed. Forty-two percent responded to a question about the maximum amount their organizations would allocate for an accreditation survey and of those, nearly all selected $1,000 as the most they could spend. Fifty-three percent of the programs selected the National Hospice Organization as their first choice to provide accreditation, and 26 percent chose JCAH. Hospital-based hospice programs selected JCAH and NHO at an even rate, but nonhospital programs selected NHO strongly over JCAH.

Following the completion of the mailed survey, the project director for the study made 17 site visits to hospice programs throughout the country to gather more in-depth information. A number of valuable insights resulted from these visits.

The project staff discovered a significant lack of understanding about JCAH in general and the hospice accreditation project in particular. Some thought the project was actually funded by NHO, whereas others had the equally false impression that NHO had no involvement at all. Many assumed that if JCAH conducted the hospice accreditation, JCAH would pay no attention to the already developed NHO standards.

It was further found that JCAH was strongly viewed by hospices as being strictly a hospital accreditation organization; it was not widely known that JCAH also surveys other heath care facilities and programs as well. The project staff found that many hospice workers were opposed to a hospital-oriented organization providing hospice accreditation, and there were strong recommendations that the JCAH survey process be modified to better accommodate home care hospices.

Hospice workers interviewed during these 17 site visits believed strongly that the JCAH process should include review of the quality of patient care during the course of any accreditation visits and that accreditation surveyors should be required to attend hospice interdisciplinary team conferences and make home visits so they would fully appreciate the depth and breadth of hospice program services. The hospice providers who were interviewed felt emphatically that accreditation should not stifle creativity and the desire to meet local needs. Each program visited by the project staff actively defended its own particular model of hospice as appropriate for the needs of its community.

As a third part of this preliminary review by JCAH, questionnaires were sent to labor unions, health insurance companies, and industrial corporations. Of the corporations, 35 percent responded and of these, only 5 percent reported having a separate section on hospice benefits in their medical insurance policies. However, about 75 percent stated they would be more likely to include hospice benefits if hospice programs were licensed by the state, 87 percent if hospice programs were accredited, and nearly 100 percent if they were demonstrated to be cost-effective. About one-half of those not currently offering hospice benefits planned to study the situation to consider whether they might do so in the future.

Of the labor unions, 12 percent responded and of these, 13 percent reported having a separate section in their medical insurance policies for hospice benefits. The union response to the rest of the questions was similar to that of the corporations.

Of the health insurance industry, 46 percent of the companies responded and of these, 2 percent reported having medical insurance policies with separate hospice benefits. Blue Cross and Blue Shield Associations reported having 19 pilot programs across the country with a total of 37 plans offering benefit coverage for hospice services.

After reviewing the three sources of information, the project staff made some additional observations. It was estimated that an average hospice program survey would require two surveyors at an average rate of $625 per day. If 150 hospice surveys were done per year, this would generate a revenue of $187,500 against projected expenses of approximately $265,000, leaving a significant deficit for any hospice accreditation efforts by JCAH. There was additional concern that many hospices would either be unable or unwilling to spend such a large amount on accreditation surveys.

The project staff also documented several accreditation and licensing activities in a number of states that might dilute a national accreditation program or at least confuse the process.

For example, the California Medical Association, working with two regional hospice associations, had written a set of hospice standards and was preparing to pilot-test a hospice accreditation survey document.[6] This project has received wide support among California hospice programs and considerable interest from a number of states that were preparing to license hospice programs or to regulate them in one fashion or another. Many of the hospices in these states expressed concern over the manner in which a national accreditation project would affect state or local efforts.

The project staff observed that the market for hospice accreditation appeared to be rather slender at that time. Although hospice workers uniformly supported the idea of setting standards and saw the need for a voluntary accreditation program, they were worried about the cost of the process. It seemed unlikely to the project staff that a hospice accreditation program would be self-supporting for some years.

They also observed that among hospice workers, JCAH was clearly the less popular choice to do the accreditation. However, it was observed that much of this feeling was probably due to a lack of information about JCAH and a false perception of it as a hospital-controlled organization.

In view of the project staff's findings and observations, a number of pertinent questions were raised for the consideration of JCAH and the advisory committee for this accreditation study. The following list summarizes most of the important policy issues concerning hospice accreditation:

- In this rapidly evolving field, will standards and accreditation programs stultify the growth and expansion of the hospice movement?
- If accreditation is timely now, who should do it, how should it be done, and within what time frame?
- How will standards and accreditation affect those states with their own activities already in motion?
- Should the NHO standards be used as the basis for hospice accreditation or is some other set of standards needed?
- Is the hospice community unified enough to be able to work cooperatively in developing acceptable standards and to support an accreditation program?
- Should only hospital-based programs be considered for accreditation at this time?
- If an accreditation program is unlikely to be self-supporting for several years, can additional funds be found to support the program in the interim?

- What is the best way to educate the community about the positive aspects of standards and accreditation?

After reviewing the data gathered during the initial investigations, the JCAH board of commissioners decided in late 1981 to work with NHO to develop a model set of standards for hospice programs that could be used as a basis for a national accreditation program. The development of a self-assessment guide and a survey guide that would become the basis for the accreditation process was also begun.

In late 1981, Peggy Falknor, the California nurse who had shepherded the initial phase of the JCAH-Kellogg project to a successful conclusion, returned to California, and Barbara McCann, a hospice administrator and social worker from New Mexico, took on the task of developing standards and a model accreditation process. A first draft of hospice standards and accreditation procedures was developed and circulated widely among hospice workers for written comments. In early 1982, six invitational conferences were held throughout the country at which hospice workers, other health care providers, and various state and local authorities were asked to discuss the standards and procedures and to offer advice for improvement.

The project staff incorporated the comments and suggestions into a second draft of standards and procedures, and in the summer of 1982, pilot tests of the proposed procedures were carried out at 19 hospice programs around the country. Hospital-based, community-based, and freestanding hospices in urban and rural areas were included in the study. Using the draft standards, a physician and a social worker-administrator, or an oncology nurse and social worker-administrator, or a social worker-administrator alone surveyed each program. The following were common observations at the 19 sites:

- Inconsistent management of physical pain and symptoms
- Inconsistent intervention by trained counselors and social workers for significant emotional problems exhibited by patients and families
- Absence of consistent spiritual services assessment and follow-up
- Inadequate or poorly trained personnel used for provision of bereavement services
- Absence of consent-for-care forms, especially in independently owned programs
- Absence of interdisciplinary team care plans signed by the attending physician
- Absence of documentation by the attending physician, team members, or the patient and family regarding nonresuscitation of a patient

The survey team was pleased that providers at all 19 sites were not surprised by the findings and were eager to learn how to improve care. The hospice workers also generally reacted favorably to the survey process and developed significantly different perceptions of JCAH as a result of participating in the project.

The experience gained in these pilot tests was fed back into the development of a final draft of the hospice standards and review procedures, which was circulated widely among hospice workers for comment and discussion. In 1983 the standards and procedures were formally adopted by JCAH and incorporated into a national accreditation program for hospices conducted by JCAH.[7,8]

JCAH Standards

At this time, the JCAH publication *Hospice Standards Manual* represents the most comprehensive and thorough document for hospice accreditation. It is also the most detailed statement of what should constitute an acceptable hospice program.

The unit of care is the patient and the patient's family or other primary caregiver. The hospice program must have a statement of patient-family rights that is available to patients and family and the public.

Care must be provided to patients and families through the means of an interdisciplinary team. These services should be available to patients and their families at home as well as in an inpatient setting. The services provided should include at least physician, nursing, psychological, social work, spiritual, and bereavement services. These services can be provided by hospice program employees, by volunteers, or through written agreements with an individual, institution, or agency. The members of the interdisciplinary team should have access to emotional support for their own needs, as well as access to in-service and continuing education programs.

Although the medical care of each patient is the responsibility of a physician, usually the patient's attending physician, the hospice program must have a medical director whose responsibilities are appropriate to the needs of the program. There must be qualified individuals to provide nursing, psychosocial, social work, spiritual, and bereavement services and to supervise the efforts of volunteer staff.

Continuity of care is an essential feature of an acceptable hospice program. This continuity must be ensured through a defined process for admission to the program, ongoing assessment of the patient-family needs, development of an interdisciplinary team care plan, and the provision of adequate patient-family information at transfer.

With regard to home care, an acceptable hospice program must ensure that home care services are available 24 hours a day, 7 days a week, particularly nursing services. Arrangements must be made for the provision of laboratory, radiology, and other services as needed at home on an emergency basis and for the availability of home health aides and homemakers as appropriate.

Hospice inpatient services must be available to all patients in the hospice program, either provided by the organization itself or through contractual arrangements with other organizations. Wherever these services are provided, there must be appropriate written policies and procedures with regard to the range of treatments that will be provided and the inpatient service's position on the resuscitation of patients. It is not necessary that hospice patients be grouped together in the same section of the inpatient facility, but there must be provision for certain hospice-characteristic features, such as patient-family privacy and accommodations for family members to remain with patients throughout the night.

There must be an accurate medical record that documents hospice program services, wherever they may be provided, and that assists in attaining continuity of care and in ensuring high-quality care.

There must be an organized governing body, or designated persons so functioning, that is responsible for establishing policy, maintaining high-quality patient-family care, and providing for management and planning of the hospice program. The hospice program must have an appropriate management and planning structure and staff, including a hospice program director appointed by the governing body or its appropriate administrative representative.

There must be an active utilization review process that monitors the allocation of hospice resources and identifies problems in the use of those resources; this utilization review process must include all services, whether provided at home or in an inpatient setting. There must also be an active quality assurance program that strives to ensure the provision of high-quality patient-family care through the monitoring and evaluation of the quality and appropriateness of hospice program services, wherever they may be delivered.

JCAH Survey Process

The JCAH survey process is organized in such a way as to ensure both fairness and accuracy and at the same time to allow some provision for individual program variations. As such, the JCAH survey procedures provide a good model for any other hospice accreditation program that might be developed by other groups or agencies.

The JCAH surveys are conducted by consultant surveyors, who are not full-time employees of JCAH and who are usually actively involved in some aspect of hospice work themselves. Most of the JCAH surveyors have had significant direct administrative or clinical experience in a hospice program, and all of them have had special training in the application of the JCAH hospice standards.

The JCAH survey ensures a program's compliance with *Hospice Standards Manual* on the basis of five sources of information: (1) statements from authorized program personnel, (2) documentation of compliance provided by program staff, (3) answers to questions or examples related to implementation of standards that allow for a judgment of compliance, (4) on-site observations by JCAH surveyors, and (5) public information interviews with consumer representatives, including staff of the program under survey.

At the completion of the on-site survey, which could range from one to three days, a summary conference is held with one or more representatives of the hospice governing body, administration, and interdisciplinary team. The surveyors present their initial findings for discussion, clarification, and correction of factual errors. Hospice program representatives are given full opportunity to comment on any adverse findings and to present clarifying information.

The decision to accredit a hospice is based on the determination that the hospice is in substantial compliance with the JCAH hospice standards; a decision to deny accreditation is based on a determination that the standards have not been complied with. A decision to deny accreditation is transmitted directly to the hospice program director and is followed by a written notice of the areas of noncompliance. The program director has the right to provide additional information and documentation to demonstrate compliance with the standards in question and is given 15 days to submit such additional material.

In addition to this opportunity to provide additional information, the hospice program director has the right to an interview with JCAH staff to further explore the deficiencies, to explain the possible reasons for deficiencies, and to identify further options with regard to accreditation at a later date. If these two additional steps are not sufficient to resolve the hospice program's disagreement with the decision to deny accreditation, the program has the right to apply for a formal hearing to appeal the decision.

In the first six weeks of the existence of the JCAH survey, only 15 applications were received, representing fewer than 1 percent of the eligible hospices.[9] This parallels a situation in which fewer than 10 percent of the nation's hospices had applied by early January 1984 for certification under the federal government's final regulations governing hospice care for Medicare recipients.[10]

California Hospice Accreditation Organization

An interest in hospice accreditation in California was fostered early in the history of hospice care in that state, with the California Medical Association, the Northern California Hospice Association, and the Hospice Organization of Southern California playing active roles in its development. In 1980, at a time when there were no other mechanisms in place for ensuring high-quality care, representatives from these groups began to develop criteria for hospice care. The criteria were refined and tested in 1982, leading to the development of draft standards of care in October 1982. In early 1983 a separate organization, the California Hospice Accreditation Organization (CHAO), was independently incorporated, and in July 1983 the CHAO board of directors approved the accreditation standards that had been developed. The approved standards subsequently have been distributed to hospice programs in California, and three pilot surveys have been done in different hospice models.

A marketing survey was mailed to hospices in California by CHAO in December 1983, asking about interest in accreditation and listing four options: (1) interested in seeking accreditation when available, (2) interested in accreditation and would like more information, (3) not interested in accreditation now but might be in the future, and (4) not interested in accreditation at all. According to a CHAO representative, responses to the marketing survey were largely in the second and third categories, indicating both interest and also hesitancy about the accreditation program offered.[11]

In general, the CHAO standards are similar in content to the JCAH standards, with the same emphasis on interdisciplinary teams, the availability of inpatient care as well as home care, documentation of all services rendered, and the existence of a quality assurance program. If there is a major difference, the California standards seem to be more flexible and to allow for more individual variation than the JCAH standards. This difference is very much in keeping with the more regional, industry-sponsored nature of the California process.

It is interesting to note that in the state just to the north of California, Oregon, an even more grass roots accreditation process has begun.[12] There the Oregon Hospice Council received a grant of $10,000 from the Episcopal Diocese to establish an accreditation process for hospices in that state. Accreditation standards were developed using the California materials, and several hospices in the state have been surveyed. The emphasis in Oregon is focused more on local standards than on other efforts around the country, and the survey process serves more as an educational and supportive review of programs than as a typical inspection and regulatory endeavor.

Major Issues in Hospice Accreditation

The central consideration in the area of hospice accreditation is the extent to which the accreditation process will dull the sense of creativity and concern that has characterized hospice programs in the United States. Hospice care has developed free of bureaucratic entanglements and dominant political forces. However, among hospice programs that began as a direct response to community needs, there is now a serious concern that reimbursement will irrevocably alter the essence of hospice care, that the shape and form of hospice programs will increasingly be determined by the third-party payer, rather than by the needs of the community. Undoubtedly, what we have referred to as the hospice movement for the past 10 years will become the hospice industry in the next five. The central challenge is the implementation of a system of accreditation that allows for diversity of methods, practices, and systems of delivery.

The importance and role of hospice accreditation becomes critical in the immediate future. Standards are the foundation of an accreditation process and the structure and content of a hospice program. In this area, a significant amount of work has been done by NHO and subsequently by JCAH. Just as the regulations for Medicare reimbursement will define a certified hospice, so too will the standards propose goals that ensure the hospice program will provide high-quality care. Accordingly, it is necessary to distinguish the differences and interrelationships between regulations and standards, particularly in light of deemed status.

Standards reflect the consensus of hospice providers as well as the current state of the art. The purpose of standards is to identify the essential characteristics of high-quality care. Regulations, on the other hand, are a more direct reflection of the political process and the minimum requirements related to specific legislative policy.

JCAH standards and HCFA draft regulations have been developed from different perspectives and, in some areas, the proposals would have a markedly different impact on a large number of hospice programs. For example, the regulations require that a hospice program provide "directly and substantially all core services, which include physician, nursing, social work, and counseling." Thus, a hospital-based program must provide inpatient care and home care; a contract with a home health agency is not allowable. The JCAH perspective views this issue as a question of care. The hospice program is responsible for ensuring continuity of care, including quality of services, regardless of the source of delivery. Thus, under JCAH standards, a hospital could contract for hospice home care services.

Inevitably, these differences will have to be worked out, but given the different perspectives of the two agencies, there may be considerable tension in the process. With JCAH focusing on quality of care and with HCFA focusing on least cost, there will doubtless be many issues that will require careful work if they are to be resolved to the satisfaction of both parties.

Duration of Accreditation

Another significant issue to hospice programs is the duration of the accreditation. JCAH is considering the merits of a one-, two-, or three-year period. Hospice services have a relatively brief track record, and many experts expect rapid change in the years ahead. From this perspective, it is clear that programs would benefit from frequent review. However, JCAH survey preparation involves significant staff time and financial resources. Hospitals, which have been subject to a standardization program since 1981 and reviewed by JCAH since 1952, have a three-year accreditation cycle. Such institutions would certainly object to an institutional review that was more frequent than is the custom at present.

An important factor in this decision is that hospitals will want to minimize the duplication of surveys; a major advantage to hospitals is that JCAH has the ability to perform simultaneous surveys. If there is a two-year cycle for hospices, then it is conceivable that a hospice survey and a hospital survey might coincide only once in a six-year period. Regardless of the outcome, it should be anticipated that the duration of the hospice accreditation cycle will change to reflect the maturity and sophistication of hospice programs.

Voluntary Accreditation

Another major issue facing JCAH is whether a hospice program housed in a hospital receives separate accreditation when surveyed. Traditionally, a "significant" service in a multiservices institution receives separate accreditation. Significance is related to the number of beds involved and the size of the budget: a psychiatric unit over 99 beds would be an example of a significant service receiving separate accreditation. Generally, hospice programs will represent a relatively insignificant segment of most hospitals on the basis of this standard.

Regardless of the size of the hospice program, however, there would always be survey questions related to the delivery of hospice services. When the program is deemed to be significant in size, a hospice-trained surveyor is added to the team. If the program is not significant in size, hospital surveyors would at least have some hospice training.

Yet, there is strong argument for requiring a hospital-based hospice program to seek separate accreditation regardless of its significance within the hospital. Separate accreditation will help to establish credibility and respectability in the traditional health care system. At this early state of development, it is important to subject hospices to scrutiny to ensure consistent standards of care. Further, if Medicare certification is sought for a hospice program, Medicare reimbursement dollars will create a separate provider and identify distinct services.

Another aspect of this issue is the effect of denying accreditation to a separate service. Under JCAH procedures, a separate service that is denied accreditation could potentially place the entire hospital accreditation in jeopardy, depending on the seriousness of the noncompliant elements such as life safety. Most likely, a contingency on the program's overall accreditation would result. Obviously, those hospitals with a hospice program that is relatively insignificant in terms of total resources put themselves at considerable risk for the sake of hospice accreditation.

Another related issue is the survey of a hospice home care program that has a contractual agreement for inpatient hospice care. In order to be accredited, the inpatient hospice care facility (be it a unit or scatter beds) will be subject to survey. If the inpatient hospice care is determined to be unsatisfactory, the question arises whether the hospital or home care agency's accreditation will be revoked because of services provided by the inpatient hospice care.

Although there are no ready answers or easy solutions, these issues highlight the interrelationship and interdependence of at least two different segments of the health care system.

The Accreditation Decision

The decision to approve or deny accreditation for a hospice facility is determined by a set of contingency criteria developed by JCAH. This is accomplished by weighting certain characteristics contained within the entire standards document. The contingency criteria represent factors that are generally considered essential to high quality hospice care, as well as some subjective value judgments as to what an achievable state of the art is at the present time. The hospice that fails to comply with these contingency criteria could be denied accreditation.

The subjective nature of these criteria has possible major ramifications. If the criteria are too stringent, many hospices may decide either to close down their programs or to continue the program and not seek accreditation. Yet the purpose of the accreditation process is particularly important to hospice care, which relies so heavily on labor-intensive high-quality care. The consultative and educational role of JCAH is particularly important in establishing a system of peer review, in which the individual patient and family will be assured of high-quality care.

When substantial compliance on a particular standard is achieved by a majority of the field, then it will no longer be used as a contingency criteria. For example, the 1982 pilot surveys established that a majority of hospice programs did not have written criteria for admission to the hospice program. As a result, as JCAH accreditation is carried out, written admission standards will be a contingency criteria because they are generally considered to be essential for patient care. When a majority of the hospice programs have accomplished this goal, it will no longer be a contingency criteria. Thus, while contingency criteria reflect the state of the art, they also represent goals toward which every hospice program strives. There is a delicate balance here between offering challenges and goals to hospice providers and simultaneously recognizing that current practice and limited resources may not make it possible for every program to achieve every goal.

Compliance

Although the JCAH survey compares a program to a perfect model, the accrediting body must also determine the extent to which an individual program must be in compliance with the given criteria to receive JCAH accreditation. The present procedure utilized in the JCAH accreditation process evaluates compliance on a continuum scale:

Substantial	Significant	Partial	Minimal	No Compliance
1	2	3	4	5

Each JCAH accrediting component determines what level of compliance constitutes satisfactory achievement. Again, these determinations must reflect the state of the art.

If the surveyor rates any of the contingency criteria lower than the predetermined number, a recommendation to correct the deficiency within a specified time is given. If the deficiency is not rectified within the time period, accreditation will be jeopardized. Although no one factor usually results in nonaccreditation, a combination of factors in the contingency criteria may clearly indicate an absence of a high quality of care. The severity of the deficiency will determine the amount of time allotted to correct the problem. Lack of a hospice bereavement program would be considered more serious than a bereavement program managed by an individual without specific training in bereavement care.

Summary

The accreditation of hospice programs may well turn out to be the determining factor in the success or failure of a nationwide system of hospice care. Clearly, a viable accreditation process requires balancing competing interests, in order to result in standards that are realistically achievable and that simultaneously require ongoing improvement in quality of care.

The danger that confronts the hospice movement as it exists today is that a new wave of caregivers will seek changes in standards previously considered essential. Yet the implementation of realistic, pragmatic accreditation standards will ensure the credibility and stability necessary for the successful delivery of hospice care throughout this country. In the absence of meaningful standards, the ultimate result will be a series of government inquiries that expose the most blatant of abuses and resolve the problems by imposing standards that may or may not be appropriate for hospice care.

In addition, a responsible accreditation program will gain the respect of important actors in the health care system. In particular, physicians and private insurance carriers who have the ability to influence attitudes of patients toward hospice care will be strongly influenced in their decision making by an active, realistic system of accreditation. Until these groups demonstrate their support of the hospice concept of care, the goal of easy access to hospice care for those in need will never become a reality.

Thus, every current provider of hospice care must stand ready to support a system of accreditation that is reliable, meaningful, and sensitive to the guiding principles of hospice care. Strong and powerful economic interests may attempt to water down the basic tenets of care by arguing that economic conditions will not allow for this or that basic service. The only way to ensure that the essence and philosophy of hospice care remain unchanged is to actively support and mold a meaningful accreditation process.

If one assumes that strong support for a viable system of accreditation exists, the subsidiary area of importance is the structure of that process. The choice will be either a national or a statewide system of accreditation. The principal advantage to a national program is the credibility that comes with a national organization applying the same standards throughout the country. It is important to point out that it is unlikely that any state accreditation program will ever receive deemed status for Medicare participation. Also, the third-party payer will be much less responsive to the hospice concept when required to interface with 50 different sets of standards as opposed to one set of standards that adjusts for regional variations. A national set of standards works best for those programs that have not yet established their financial stability and credibility within the community. Meeting the standards is a threshold achievement that forms a new base of stability for the organization to build on.

At the same time there is a fear, particularly among community-based hospice providers, that national standards will not be responsive to regional, local, or rural needs. Some concern exists that a large, national accreditation body could run roughshod over a small, less powerful component. This perspective would encourage the development of state programs as a way of avoiding possible confrontation with a group that is seen to have interests that conflict with those of the hospice movement.

The simple reality is that in the pluralistic hospice field, both types of accreditation will, and probably should, exist. In those states where hospice care has a long history, state accreditation programs will serve actively to educate and represent the interests of participating programs before private and national bodies that monitor hospice care.

Hospice providers that are wary of national accreditation should recognize that a national process generates resources sufficient to recruit surveyors with sensitivity and experience in the new type of program to be surveyed. The standards are written to be applied, and it takes an expert to make the judgment as to whether a particular program complies with the theoretical model. Accrediting agencies are in the business of judging a program on its merits, not on the literal interpretation of a given standard.

References

1. International Work Group on Death, Dying, and Bereavement. Assumptions and principles underlying standards for terminal care. *American Journal of Nursing.* 1979 Feb.

2. Foster, Z. Standards for hospice care: Assumptions and principles. *Health and Social Work.* 1979. 4:117-28.

3. National Hospice Organization. *Standards of a Hospice Program of Care,* 6th revision. McLean, VA: NHO, 1979.

4. National Hospice Organization. *Revised Principles and Standards of Hospice Care.* Arlington, VA: NHO, 1981.

5. Falknor, H. P., and Kugler, D. JCAH hospice project, interim report: Phase I. Mimeo, Joint Commission on Accreditation of Hospitals, Chicago, 1981 July.

6. Hospice accreditation criteria, preliminary working draft. Mimeo, Bay Area Hospice Association (San Francisco)-California Medical Association-Southern California Hospice Association, San Francisco, 1982 June 18.

7. Joint Commission on Accreditation of Hospitals. *Hospice Standards Manual.* Chicago: JCAH, 1983.

8. Joint Commission on Accreditation of Hospitals. *Hospice Self-Assessment and Survey Guide.* Chicago: JCAH, 1983.

9. Beresford, L. Certification, accreditation, and licensing. *California Hospice Report,* 1984 March. 2(3):7.

10. Only 21 hospices apply for Medicare certification under HHS' new rules. *Hospital Week.* 1984 Jan. 13. 20(2):2.

11. Accreditation: A tale of two programs. *California Hospice Report.* 1984 March. 2(3):6.

12. Accreditation experience in other states. *California Hospice Report.* 1984 March. 2(3):11.

Chapter 7

Evaluation of Hospice Programs

Jeffrey Wales, Ph.D.

Since 1967, when St. Christopher's Hospice was established in London, there has been a strong and steady growth in the number of hospices available to care for the dying. In 1974, the first hospice in the United States was opened in New Haven, Connecticut. Today, it is estimated that there are more than 1,000 hospice programs in existence, with more being planned all the time.

This rapid growth of hospice programs has been fueled by the assumption that hospice provides superior care to those dying of cancer.[1-6] Compared with conventional care, it is believed that the hospice is more effective at controlling a patient's pain, providing a secure and caring environment, and helping the patient's relatives through the difficult period of bereavement. Such humane care seems a welcome relief from traditional care, which is seen as treating the dying patient as a nonperson or a failure of modern medicine.

Whether to provide hospice care hardly seems an issue anymore. Nearly everyone is a proponent of the programs: patients, family members, doctors, nurses, hospital administrators, government officials, and even insurance company representatives. Can there be any real doubt that hospice care is better than conventional care?

Yes, there are significant doubts, and for a very simple reason: the relative effectiveness of hospice care has yet to be scientifically proven. There is very little in the scientific literature that bears on the question of hospice effectiveness and cost. Much has been written about hospices, but thus far there has not been a single major scientific study that has randomly assigned patients to hospice care and traditional care and compared the two groups for differences in the cost and effectiveness of care received. Until randomized control trials are conducted, the question of whether the hospice does indeed provide better care can only be answered by the impressions of hospice client groups. Such impressions, unfortunately, constitute shaky grounds on which to base decisions affecting the expenditure of millions of scarce health care dollars.

Consequently, there is a need to thoroughly appraise the performance and cost of hospice programs, using accepted procedures of scientific evaluation. Carefully designed evaluations of hospice programs must be carried out and the results rigorously analyzed, to see that the subjective impressions of hospice are confirmed by objective studies.

This chapter will:

- Discuss why it is important to evaluate hospice studies
- Review current hospice evaluation studies
- Outline the model for the evaluation of the Veterans Administration Wadsworth Hospice being conducted by the UCLA School of Medicine
- Discuss problems of conducting an evaluation in an ongoing hospital setting
- Offer suggestions of how to further explore hospice evaluation

The Value of Hospice Evaluations

A thorough evaluation is composed of the following four major parts based on core questions addressed by the evaluation:[7]

- Program planning. What is the extent and distribution of the target population? Is the program designed in conformity with its intended goals, and are chances of successful implementation maximized?
- Program monitoring. Is the program reaching the people to whom it is addressed? Is the program providing the resources, services, or other benefits intended in the research design?
- Impact assessment. Is the program effective in achieving intended goals? Can the results of the program be explained by some alternate process that does not include the program? Is the program having some effects that were not intended?
- Economic efficiency. What are the costs to deliver services and benefits to program participants? Is the program an efficient use of resources compared with alternative uses?

A thorough, scientific hospice evaluation offers several distinct advantages over incomplete approaches. First, it defines and clarifies a hospice's organization, structure, and processes. Second, it offers valid and reliable data on overall hospice effectiveness. Third, it identifies which of a hospice's several components (for example, inpatient care, home care, consultation service, or volunteer program) are more effective than the others.

Fourth, it provides data on how much it costs to operate a hospice relative to other forms of comparable care, how much of the total hospice budget is consumed by any given component, and, in some cases, how much of an increment in effectiveness can be purchased per dollar expended. Finally, a complete hospice evaluation will often achieve unintended advantages such as improved record keeping and the facilitation of better communication among members of the hospice staff as well as between the hospice staff and other parts of the hospital. Each of these will be discussed in turn.

Program Clarification

The rapidly advancing hospice movement has left in its wake a trail of organizations that are called hospices but that often vary considerably among themselves. In the United States, at least three major models of hospice care can be delineated.[8] They are (1) the freestanding model (examples include Hospice, Incorporated of New Haven, Connecticut, and the Hill Haven Hospice in Tucson, Arizona), (2) the institution-affiliated model (such as the hospice unit in the Kaiser-Permanente Hospital in Hayward, California, and the V.A. Wadsworth Medical Center hospice in Los Angeles), and (3) the community-based hospice, or the "hospice without walls" (including the Hospice/Hospital Home Health Care Agency of Torrance, California, and the Hospice of Marin, Marin County, California). Each of these models varies on such factors as means of finance, the number and type of services offered, mean charges for services, and the composition of the staff.[9]

With such wide variation among hospices, an important question arises: What is the difference between hospice and nonhospice? If a model of a hospice showing its goals, organization, daily activities, staffing patterns, and physical facilities were to be developed, and if that model were to be compared with a comparable model of conventional care for the terminally ill cancer patient, how different would the two models be? With some varieties of hospice, the differences would likely be clear. With other varieties, one may be hard pressed to detect significant differences.

It is important to make such a comparison, because the desired outcomes of hospice care — pain control, patient-family satisfaction, freedom from depression — may be achieved only in some varieties and not in others, or the different hospices may be effective in certain areas and not in others. Furthermore, those in a position of designing a hospice, funding it, or reimbursing it for services rendered must know where traditional cancer care leaves off and where hospice care begins.

A thorough, scientific evaluation can help with this problem. First, a model is developed for both hospice and conventional care models. These models are written descriptions of a hospice's structure and process. *Structure* refers to the physical and organizational attributes of the care mode, such as the number of beds and the number and type of staff positions required per X number of patients. *Process* refers to the activities that must be performed by the various staff members to successfully reach the goals of that particular mode of care (for example, a clinical protocol).

Second, these models are compared with one another to determine how hospice care is like other modes of care and how it is different. As an additional step, the outcomes of the two modes of care can be measured and evaluated to determine if one mode is more effective than the other in reaching such typical hospice goals as pain control, satisfaction with care, and reduced anxiety. If one shows the desired outcomes and the other does not, presumably this is caused by the better design of the successful model's structure and processes.

In this way, hospice planners, administrators, funding agencies, and evaluators are provided with specific written criteria of effective hospice structure and process, against which they may compare the structure and process attributes of the many programs that identify themselves as hospices.

Such criteria provide powerful tools for those who are determined to expend health care resources only on those hospice programs that promise to do the most good in the most cost-effective way. In addition, the criteria provide a way of establishing standards of organizational performance for all new hospices. Such standards could result in meaningful accreditation or licensure procedures administered by local, state, or national governments or by such organizations as the National Hospice Organization (NHO).

Measurement of Hospice Effectiveness

The most important advantage of hospice evaluation is that it provides decision makers with a report card on hospice effectiveness. The National Hospice Organization in its *Standards of a Hospice Program of Care* (Nov. 1981) states that "the purpose of a hospice is to provide support and care for persons in the last phases of disease so that they can live as fully and comfortably as possible." This philosophy, in turn, is translated into specific goals or objectives, including controlling pain, increasing satisfaction with the care received, lessening depression and anxiety, and supporting surviving family members through bereavement. The question is this: Is the hospice better at reaching these goals than conventional care?

A search of the hospice literature reveals a plethora of anecdotal data on the superiority of hospice care. Letters from surviving family members are frequently quoted. Individual, subjective self-congratulations from hospice staff members about the quality of their own work exist in great numbers. Hopeful statements from hospice program proponents are available from family and staff.

Although letters from family members and staff testimonials are important, they cannot in themselves answer the question of hospice effectiveness. Such information frequently is not valid, reliable, or representative and therefore may be of questionable value.

This point is illustrated by a consideration of the goals of a hospice planner and how the lack of valid and reliable data may affect the ability to reach those goals. A hospice planner tries to develop a model that (1) is capable of delivering the care for which it was designed, (2) is cost-effective, and (3) is transferable to other settings. Hospice planners and staff attempt to reach these goals by trying different mixes of funding, staffing, physical facilities, and patient loads. Which mix works best can only be known through careful feedback in the form of valid and reliable data. Trying to develop and administer a high quality, cost-effective hospice without such data is like trying to drive a car with a faulty steering mechanism.

Data are valid when the scales selected or developed to measure a variable such as pain or depression do in fact measure that variable and not another one. For example, one of the goals of hospice is to prevent or reduce depression. Depression is a complex phenomenon that requires a thoroughly tested scale (a series of carefully selected questions) that will actually discriminate among those people who have depression and those who do not and, for those who do, determine the degree to which they suffer from it. Data are reliable when the scale used to measure depression produces the same score at two different times (assuming that there has been no change in the actual depression in that period). Finally, data are representative when they come from all the constituencies of the hospice, not just from those that are most convenient. It may be that an administrator's image of how well the hospice is doing comes from a very small number of staff with whom he or she feels a rapport. If they are all enthusiastic supporters of the hospice, but there are other staffers or patients who harbor complaints, the administrator's view of the success of the hospice will be biased. Unless the various constituencies are scientifically identified and sampled, biases in the results can be assumed, and manipulation of the hospice program to a more effective goal attainment is not likely.

Of the various goals of scientific evaluation, the most important is trying to produce valid, reliable, and representative data so that an objective evaluation of hospice effectiveness can be made. Most of the detailed work that goes on in an evaluation is to this end.

Assessment of Hospice Components

A hospice is often composed of several components, such as the inpatient unit, a home-care program, and a volunteer service. In addition, goals range from specific, medically oriented ones such as controlling pain and relieving symptoms, to broad, unspecific ones such as lending dignity to the patient's dying days. It would be naive to assume that all components of a hospice program are performing equally well (or poorly) in all circumstances or that all hospice goals are being reached at the same pace. It is no easy task to determine which components perform well, yet it would be valuable to know this.

Because health care dollars are limited, being able to assess the relative effectiveness of various components of a hospice would serve hospice planners' goals well. It may be that one would want disproportionately more of the limited funds to go toward those components that are proven effective and to encourage the development of those kinds of services. Or, as an opposite strategy, one might wish to put disproportionately more toward those components that are performing poorly in hopes of improving them for a stronger overall hospice program.

A thorough scientific evaluation can provide this information. As an example, consenting cancer patients might be randomly assigned to either the experimental group (hospice) or the control group (other wards in the hospital). Once in the hospice, patients either become inpatients or home care patients (assuming that the hospice has these two components in its program). Accordingly, control patients become either inpatients or outpatients. By interviewing patients in both groups and comparing the scale scores of hospice inpatients with hospice home care patients, investigators may be able to elicit something meaningful about the relative effectiveness of these two hospice components. By comparing hospice inpatients to control inpatients or hospice home care patients with control outpatients, investigators may be able to speak to the effectiveness of the various hospice components relative to comparable components outside the hospice.

Cost Determination

In these days of limited resources and increased accountability, there is much interest in cost analyses. Such analyses are often an integral part of an evaluation study and can offer invaluable information to hospice program planners and administrators.

In a randomized control trial, it is possible to tally all the costs of caring for hospice and control patients, whether such costs are apparent (such as drugs and laboratory costs) or not (such as days lost from work by spouse or other family members caring for the patient). The cost of care for the two groups can then be compared to determine if there are significant differences. In this way, valid and reliable data are produced on how much it costs to operate a hospice relative to other forms of care, how much of the total hospice budget is consumed by any given component of it and, when combined with other noncost measures (such as pain reports and satisfaction with care received), how much of an increment in effectiveness can be purchased per dollar expended.

Data such as these perhaps more than any other will likely determine the future course of hospice development in the United States. As the movement matures and hospices become institutionalized, issues of cost accounting will play an ever greater role. Those organizations that have thorough cost data for their hospice operations will surely be in a better position to deal with the politics of program continuation and funding than those that do not.

Unintended Advantages

Because the evaluation staff interacts frequently with hospice staff regarding sources of data and how to interpret those data, many suggestions arise for improving data collection techniques. This interaction may lead to a more efficient operation after the evaluation is complete.

In addition, the hospice evaluation staff usually speaks with all sectors of the hospice staff, including the director, chaplains, pharmacists, doctors, nurses, and housekeeping staff. These discussions tend to result in more frequent communication among hospice staff members. Hospice evaluators must also deal with staff in the large hospital with which the hospice may be affiliated. This contact tends to increase communication between hospice staff and staff in the large hospital to the benefit of both.

Hospice Evaluation Studies — A Review

With advantages such as these, it would be expected that there are many studies to which one could look for guidance, but this is not the case. The hospice movement is so new that there has not been enough time to accumulate a body of evaluation literature; also, such studies are expensive and can be difficult to do. However, certain generalizations of hospice evaluation literature can be made.

First, studies are mostly anecdotal and descriptive rather than experimental; that is, most of them lack a sound research design. Therefore, the data must be considered not valid, unreliable, and biased. Second, there is too much attention to hospice structure and process and not enough to outcomes; there are many studies in the literature that describe how a hospice is organized, developed, and operated but very few that speak to the issue of how well a hospice does what it is intended to do. Third, many of the existing studies have been done by hospice staff, even though the staff does not have the time to offer care and do research as well, was not trained to do rigorous scientific research, and, as staff, has a vested interest in proving the effectiveness of its program. Finally, existing studies cover some issues well (such as how satisfied patients are with hospice care) but avoid other equally important issues (such as the cost of providing care relative to conventional care), probably because of the strong assumption at the start among hospice workers that hospice offers superior care.

There are, however, a handful of hospice impact assessment studies done by evaluation researchers. These studies, summarized below, offer a glimpse of the issues raised and the methods employed to study them.

Hinton[10] studied a group of 80 married persons with malignant neoplasms and a prognosis of no more than three months, to determine whether those who were receiving hospice care were less anxious, depressed, and angry than those receiving care in a general hospital ward. The patients had an average age of 58 years, were matched on age, sex, religion, and the time between the assessment and the patient's death. On average, they were interviewed approximately 10 weeks before death. He found that hospice patients were less depressed and anxious than others and preferred more open communication about their illness.

Parkes,[11] using a sample of 55 spouses of patients who died at St. Christopher's Hospice in London and a group of 34 spouses of patients who had not received hospice care, sought to determine whether hospice patients were less reluctant to be admitted for treatment, reported less pain, and whether they were more likely to be aware of their prognosis. Results supported his hypotheses.

In a follow-up study, Parkes[12,13] asked the surviving spouses to make self-assessments of their own reactions to the type of care provided to them and the patients at St. Christopher's Hospice and at other hospitals in the vicinity. He learned that spouses of patients at St. Christopher's were far more likely to spend more time at the patient's bedside than those at other hospitals. In addition, he found that the spouses of patients at St. Christopher's were less worried than others by the need to conceal their own fears from the patient.

Barzelai[14] studied a sample of 24 surviving family members to learn of patients' pain and the family members' access to information about the patient's condition. By using a mailed questionnaire for this group (there was no control group), he learned that 82 percent of the family members thought that the now-deceased patient had had his pain relieved and that 80 percent of them felt that they had had adequate information on the patient's condition at that time.

Silver[15] identified various dimensions of care, such as health and medical care, pain and comfort care, social and spiritual care, and both patient and family emotional care and found that, in general, patients demonstrated greater improvement in all dimensions with increased length of stay in the hospice program. Because there was no control group, it is not possible to conclude that this improvement was due to the hospice program alone. In addition, data were collected only from the family members and not from the patients themselves.

Van de Creek[16] queried the families of all the first year's patients (n = 70) at the Hospice of Columbus, Ohio, and reported that more than 90 percent of the 64 percent who responded were satisfied with the services rendered, but only 75 percent were satisfied with the physicians. There was no control group, and responses were from one time only.

One study, sponsored by the National Cancer Institute[17] and conducted by the Kaiser-Permanente Health Plan in Los Angeles, has been concluded. It was a wide-ranging descriptive study that attempted to determine the appropriateness and transferability of the British model of hospice and to examine the implementation of the hospice concept in different medical milieus — specifically, a freestanding hospice within a health maintenance organization (Kaiser-Permanente), a freestanding hospice within a hospital (Riverside in Boonton, New Jersey), and a freestanding hospice associated with a long-term care program (Hill Haven in Tucson, Arizona). It also compared the cost of service provided across the three hospices and developed more specific questions concerning the spending patterns, the role of hospice and its impact on the family, and utilization of individual services.

The largest hospice evaluation study to date includes 26 hospices around the country and is being conducted by the School of Medicine at Brown University with financial support from the Health Care Financing Administration, the Robert Wood Johnson Foundation, and the John A. Hartford Foundation.[18,19] It is a quasi-experimental study designed to answer four major questions:

- What is the differential impact of hospice on the quality of life of terminally ill patients and their families as compared to conventional or customary care?
- What are the differential costs of caring for comparable terminally ill patients in hospices and in customary care settings?
- What is the likely impact of Medicare reimbursement on the organizational structure, staffing pattern, and cost of hospices?
- What would be the likely national utilization cost of hospice care if Medicare and Medicaid coverage were broadened to include hospice care?

This major study is designed to provide a data base for future federal fiscal policy for reimbursement of hospice care.

Another major hospice evaluation study has just been completed, this one sponsored by the American Cancer Society and conducted by the University of California at Los Angeles School of Medicine, with the author as project director.[20] It dealt with the hospice program at the Wadsworth Veterans Administration Hospital in Los Angeles and is the only hospice evaluation study to date that utilizes the randomized controlled trial design. The study design is described below.

UCLA Model of a Scientific Hospice Evaluation Study

To choose a single model to represent the method for hospice program evaluation is difficult, because there are many ways to do an evaluation. Thus, it is necessary to more narrowly define the conditions under which the model applies.

First, of the major classes of evaluation activities described by Rossi, Freeman, and Wright,[21] the focus is on the impact assessment model, because this is the one that best addresses the question of how well the hospice does what it does (that is, how much impact is it having on its target population?). Models that address program planning, program monitoring, and cost-effectiveness are also important, but they entail separate methodologies, and a thorough description of each is beyond the scope of this chapter. The impact assessment model was chosen for description here because it focuses on the crucial question of hospice performance and because its methodology is complex and worthy of examination. However, the UCLA study described below contains parts of each of the above four models described by Rossi and others, and each will be discussed when relevant.

Second, there are a number of designs that can be used to measure impact. Campbell and Stanley[22] classify them as preexperimental, quasi-experimental, and experimental. The randomized controlled trial, an experimental design, is considered the best for program impact evaluation because it controls more sources of bias than any other and hence offers the best validity.[23-25] The University of California at Los Angeles Hospice Evaluation Study successfully employed such a design.

Third, with regard to a hospice's impact, the question arises of impact on whom or what. The impact can be on the hospice patients themselves, their family members, the hospice staff, the larger hospital of which the hospice may be a part, or the community at large. For our purpose, the focus is on the hospice patients themselves as well as their family members.

The UCLA evaluation effort is organized into a number of logical steps, each of which is discussed in turn:

1. Identify hospice goals and define them in operational terms
2. Select or develop scales to measure variables
3. Develop a research design
4. Determine the sample of respondents
5. Develop a protocol for data collection
6. Collect data
7. Perform the analyses

8. Write the report summarizing the findings and make policy change recommendations to appropriate decision makers

Identify Hospice Goals and Define Them in Operational Terms

Most organizations tend to have global and imprecise goals, and the hospice program is no exception. For example, perhaps the single most important goal in the hospice is to provide a caring environment so that the seriously ill cancer patient can die with peace and dignity. Although this goal is laudable, its imprecision makes it difficult to determine whether the hospice is successful at providing such an environment. It is necessary to state a series of more modest, specific goals, which when taken together provide an environment conducive to a peaceful and dignified death.

For example, if patients are to be provided with a dignified death, they must be freed from intense pain and insofar as possible the debilitating and often embarrassing symptoms of their disease. Therefore, a subgoal can be stated as follows: patients will be given pain medication at regular intervals to completely control their pain. By breaking global goals down into their parts, evaluators can measure the subgoals. It is difficult to measure directly the degree to which a meaningful environment has been provided for a person's dying process, but it is possible to determine whether terminal cancer patients have been put on a consistent pain control regimen using whatever drugs are necessary to completely control their pain. Further, one can interview both hospice and nonhospice patients about their pain to determine whether hospice patients report less pain and fewer symptoms.

To list the subgoals in logical order and in such a way that they are both measureable and related to the global goals, evaluators must sit down with hospice staff members for thorough discussions. The hospice staff members state the goals as they see them, and the evaluator attempts to structure those goals in such a way as to satisfy the requirements for adequate measurement.

For the UCLA-Wadsworth VA Hospice Evaluation, such meetings resulted in a list of 13 goals:
1. To free the patient of pain and unpleasant symptoms
2. To spare the patient unnecessary diagnostic procedures
3. To facilitate home stays for those who desire to be at home
4. To increase the patient's and family's satisfaction with the care received
5. To involve the family members and the patient with decisions made about the patient's care
6. To help the patient and family with legal, economic, bureaucratic, and spiritual problems associated with terminal illness and death

7. To lessen the negative psychological effects, such as depression and anxiety, suffered by the patient and family as they face the reality of death and dying
8. To lessen the ill effects of bereavement for the grieving family
9. To provide a mechanism for relieving staff stress
10. To strive to deliver hospice care to those patients targeted as most likely to benefit from such care
11. To educate other health care providers about hospice concepts
12. To instill in the patient and family a sense of continuity of hospice care throughout the illness regardless of the circumstances of the patient
13. To ensure that the responsibility for the patient's care is borne by the entire hospice team rather than just by one or two staff members

After the goals have been identified, it is necessary to list the specific variables needing measurement. For example, for the goal of controlling the pain and symptoms of the dying cancer patient, it is necessary to measure pain and symptoms. In like fashion, for the goal of lessening the negative psychological effects suffered by the patients and their families, it might be necessary to measure patient and family depression and anxiety, as well as the level of morbidity among family members during bereavement.

Select or Develop Scales to Measure Variables

The next task is to decide how each of the variables will be measured. If one wants to know whether hospice patients suffer less pain than non-hospice patients, it is necessary to determine how much pain each type of patient has. Unfortunately, pain is a complex phenomenon, and measuring its existence and degree is no easy task. Simply asking a patient whether he or she is in pain and to what extent is often not adequate for scientific measurement. Because different persons have different ideas about what pain is and how incapacitating it is to them, a scale must be developed that allows the investigator to be reasonably sure that the patients who are being asked about their pain have similar notions about what pain is.

An example of such a scale is the Melzack Pain Questionnaire (MSQ), developed by Ronald Melzack in Canada and used in the UCLA Hospice Evaluation Study.[26] It consists of a pain rating index, three major classes of descriptive words (sensory, affective, and evaluative) by which patients specify subjective pain experience, and several items that determine the properties of the pain experience.

Unlike pain and anxiety, the measurement of other variables may be very straightforward and may not require the use of any scales or intermediary measurement procedures. For example, to obtain a measurement of the number of home care visits to a hospice patient, it may only be necessary to review the patient's record and actually count the number of such visits. It may be necessary to clearly describe or define a home visit, but once that definition is laid down, no scales are necessary for its measurement.

Occasionally, scales are not available for the measurement of certain variables, and they must actually be constructed by the researchers doing the evaluation. In this case, the scales must meet rigorous standards of validity and reliability, so that the results can be compared with other available data and can be duplicated by others. (See the work of Ware, Snyder, and Wright for further useful insights into this problem.[27]) It is usually more efficient to use already existing scales, if possible.

Develop a Research Design

Once the hospice goals have been specified and scales selected to measure relevant variables, a research design must be worked out. "A research design is the arrangement of conditions for collection and analysis of data in a manner that aims to combine relevance to the research purpose with economy in procedure."[28] It follows that different purposes would require different research designs. Indeed, there is a wide array of designs for evaluation research. Although preexperimental and quasi-experimental designs are popular in such research, they tend to be weak designs because they are relatively less effective at controlling biases such as the differential selection of respondents from comparison groups.[29] Despite the inability of most of these designs to control many sources of bias, they are able to control some of them and they represent a step forward from simply using ad hoc, nonscientific methods.

The model presented here, however, is based on the randomized control trial (RCT) experimental design (see figure 1, below).

$$
\begin{array}{llccc}
 & & t_1 & & t_2 \\
E & R & O_1 & \times & O_2 \\
C & R & O_1 & & O_2
\end{array}
$$

E = Experimental (hospice) group
C = Control (conventional care) group
R = Random assignment of respondents to experimental or control conditions
O = Observation (in this model, an interview of patients or significant others regarding pain and symptoms, psychological state, or satisfaction with care)
X = Experimental treatment (hospice care)
t_1 = First point in time (prior to the experimentals receiving hospice care)
t_2 = Second point in time (after experimentals receive hospice care)

Figure 1. Randomized Control Trial Design for Hospice Evaluation

Because the RCT design controls so many sources of bias, it offers strong internal validity and therefore represents the preeminent design in evaluation research.[30-32] This design enhances the chance of obtaining quality data by providing baseline measures, a control group of nonhospice cancer patients against which to measure the experimental hospice effects, and the elimination of systematic bias through randomization.

In the UCLA study, the hospice experimental treatment is variously defined as efforts to control pain, reduce depression, or enhance satisfaction with care. Because the patients are interviewed periodically from the time of admission to the study until death, the design is modified as in figure 2, below.

$$
\begin{array}{llcccccc}
 & & t_1 & & t_2 & & t_3 & & t_x \\
E & R & 0_1 & \times & 0_2 & \times & 0_3 & \times & 0_x \\
C & R & 0_1 & & 0_2 & & 0_3 & & 0_x \\
\end{array}
$$

Figure 2. UCLA Study Research Design

Determine the Sample of Respondents

The next step is to determine from whom data will be collected. Because hospice goals indicate that those helped and supported are primarily patients and their families, it is necessary to interview both patients and family members. The question is: which ones to interview?

In the UCLA study, the decision was made to try to interview all hospice-eligible patients and their families within the Veterans Administration Wadsworth Medical Center. The term *hospice-eligible* refers to those who have a confirmed cancer diagnosis and a prognosis of approximately six months. To identify these patients and their family members, a systematic search of the hospital was conducted to determine all hospice-eligible patients. Once the initial list had been compiled, a continuing effort was made throughout the entire data-collection period to identify each new patient who qualified as hospice-eligible. Once the patients were identified, their attending physicians were consulted to determine the acceptability of each patient for possible referral to the hospice for participation in the study. Those patients deemed appropriate were approached by hospice evaluation staff using standard informed-consent documents and asked to participate in the study. Those who consented to participate (92 percent of those eligible) were randomly assigned to the hospice or to conventional care. If assigned to hospice, they were physically transferred to the hospice; if to conventional care, they were left in their present place of care. For all the consenting patients who had a family member (63 percent), the family member was approached and also asked to participate.

Of this group, 95 percent participated.

Develop a Protocol for Data Collection

The next question to decide is how and when to collect relevant data. There are two data collection phases: one is to organize the content and form of the interview schedule, and the other is to determine the schedule of interview administrations.

In the first phase, how many interview schedules will be needed and which scales will go in which interview schedules must be determined. Three interview schedules were used for the UCLA study. Two of them were for the patients. The first contained the pain and symptoms scales. The second contained scales that measure psychological-state variables such as depression and anxiety, as well as scales that measure several satisfaction variables, including satisfaction with the care received, the environment, and involvement in care. Two schedules were used because of the necessity to interview patients more frequently about their pain than about their psychological state or satisfaction.

In the second phase, a schedule of interview administrations must be developed. How often and when to give an interview depends on several factors, including the variability of the phenomenon being measured as well as how long a patient is expected to live. Because pain is likely to vary more often than a patient's satisfaction with his environment, it was necessary to schedule pain interviews fairly frequently. In the UCLA study, they were scheduled for the time of admission to the study, then once a week for the first month, followed by biweekly interviews until the death of the patient. The interviews containing the scales for psychological state and satisfaction for patients and family members were given at the time of the patient's admission to the study; 7, 21, and 42 days later; and monthly thereafter until the death of the patient.

Collect Data

Data collection runs for a certain period of time based on how many patients are necessary for the sample.

The question of determining the number of subjects required for any given study is a complex one and beyond the scope of this chapter. Suffice it to say that the analysis anticipated for this evaluation required 250 patients. Checking the average number of referrals to the hospice over a period of time, it was determined that a little over three terminal cancer patients per week were being identified and referred. At that rate, it would take approximately 18 months to reach a sample size of 250. The size of the family member sample was determined by the number of family members available within this sample of 250 patients. In the UCLA study, that number turned out to be 157, or 63 percent of the size of the patient sample.

Perform the Analyses

Once the data have been collected from the respondents and the proper sample size has been reached, the data must be analyzed in such a way as to allow the investigator to answer the question of whether the hospice provides significantly better care in the areas of pain relief, reduced depression, satisfaction, and so on. A detailed discussion of the various statistical techniques for doing such analyses is not the present purpose of this chapter, but the logic of the analyses is briefly outlined.

Each respondent, whether a patient or a significant other, will have a score on every variable measured for each time he or she is interviewed. For example, suppose every patient who entered the study lived exactly one month more from that time. In a hypothetical case such as this, each patient respondent would have had four pain interviews (one at admission and once per week for that month). Because there is one scale within the interview to measure pain and one to measure symptoms, the patient has two scores for each of the four interviews. With data such as these, it is possible to construct a plot with the week of the interview on the horizontal axis and the patient's pain scale score on the vertical axis for both hospice and control patients (see figure 3, below).

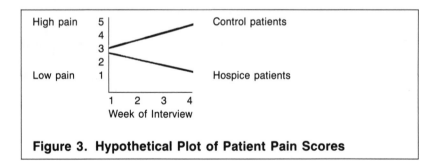

Figure 3. Hypothetical Plot of Patient Pain Scores

If these were real data, the plot would show that both hospice and control patients were experiencing a similar pain level upon being admitted to the study. (This would be expected because of the random assignment of terminal cancer patients to the hospice or control groups.) But over time, control patients' pain increases; hospice patients' pain decreases. The decrease for hospice patients is presumably due to the superiority of the hospice pain-control regimen.

When the data warrant it, statistical models can be used to determine whether the difference in pain scores between hospice and control patients at any given time or at all times is significant, that is, whether the difference is due to factors other than chance.

This same basic analysis strategy can be performed for the scores on all dependent variables studied in the hospice impact assessment.

Write the Final Report

The final step is to interpret the data and organize them in such a way as to answer the research questions posed at the beginning of the evaluation. For example, do hospice patients suffer less pain than their conventional-care counterparts? To answer this question, one or more plots of hospice and control patients' pain scores can be presented and interpreted. The plot might look like figure 4, below.

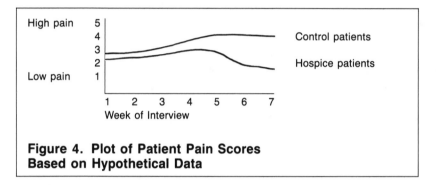

Figure 4. Plot of Patient Pain Scores Based on Hypothetical Data

According to the data in figure 4, the answer would be yes, hospice patients would suffer less pain than control patients. However, the difference does not appear until after the third week (probably because it takes that long for the newly initiated hospice pain-control regimen to take effect), and the difference does not become a significant one until the seventh week. (This statement assumes that significance tests have been performed and reported.)

In like manner, each of the originally posed research questions can be reviewed and answered in turn.

Although the specific content of a report will vary depending on its purpose and its intended audience, in general it will include information on the methods used in the evaluation (such as which research design and which scales were used), a description of the sample (such as the diagnosis of the patients and the income, sex, and occupation of the patients and family members interviewed) so that the reader can determine the types of patients to which the findings might apply and, on occasion, the policy implications of the findings.

An example of a policy implication can be drawn from the hypothetical plot in figure 4, which indicates that the difference in pain scores is not significant until the seventh week. If the median survival time for the hospice is five weeks, then most hospice patients will not have their pain controlled any more effectively than those in conventional care. One way to correct this problem is to recruit terminal cancer patients to the hospice earlier than heretofore, keeping in mind that there are problems with this approach, too, such as the increased difficulty of determining hospice-eligibility (namely, a terminal prognosis) earlier in the course of the disease.

Problems with Randomized Control Trial Hospice Evaluations

Designing research carefully is a challenge. Conducting such research within the boundaries of a large and complex organization (such as a hospital) is perhaps the greater challenge. The challenge is to remain true to the guidelines of a carefully designed evaluation project and at the same time to cope with the strictures imposed from the daily routines of the organization in which the evaluation is taking place. Four major problem areas will be addressed here as examples of the kinds of difficulties evaluators may face.[33] The four problems are (1) disruption of the normal hospital routine, (2) emergence of ethical dilemmas, (3) rise in territorial jealousies, and (4) lowered hospice patient census.

Disruption of Normal Routine

The imposition of an experimental research design interrupts normal lines of referral. Prior to the UCLA study, physicians referred their patients to the hospice directly. When the study began, it became necessary for all referrals to go through the research team. Because referrals who consented to participate in the study would be randomly assigned to either hospice or conventional care, a physician's referral to the hospice would not necessarily result in the patient's being placed within the hospice. Such a situation can be seen as a restriction in a physician's autonomy or even a limitation on the physician's ability to treat the patient as he or she sees fit.

However, the reality of the situation was that the number of referrals to the hospice was always higher than the capacity of the hospice, with the result that prior to the study many referred patients would not have been admitted to the hospice. The net effect of the study was to cause those who did enter the hospice to get there by way of chance rather than by previous referral patterns. Careful education of medical personnel prior to the start of randomization mitigated the disruption caused by this research procedure.

Emergence of Ethical Dilemmas

An experimental design with random assignment of patients and significant others to the experimental or control groups raises several ethical problems. The most important concerns the denial of experimental treatment (hospice care) to at least three groups of patients: (1) those patients who have agreed to participate in the study but who were randomly assigned to the control group, (2) those who are unwilling to participate in the study but who might have otherwise accepted hospice care, and (3) those who are unable to give informed consent due to physical or mental limitations. Denial of treatment to such groups is an inevitable consequence of a randomized trial design. Technically speaking, however, the effectiveness of the hospice concept is unproven; therefore, it can be argued that the denial of this service, coupled with the fact that conventional care is readily available, makes this less of an ethical problem than it may at first appear to be. However, even though the hospice concept is technically unproven, hospice care is popular and sought after by patients and their family members, thereby keeping the ethical dilemma at the forefront.

Prior to the start of randomization, many patients were denied hospice treatment because of the limited capacity of the hospice relative to the number of referrals received. The choice of which referral patient should be admitted to the inpatient unit depended on the collective judgment of the hospice staff. Patients with physical or mental problems serious enough to cause hospice staff to question whether the hospice treatment would be effective were denied admission in favor of those believed to be more responsive to external stimuli. With the advent of randomization, the hospice staff no longer had control over which patients were admitted to the hospice. However, and most important, the total number of patients receiving hospice care did not change.

Rise in Territorial Jealousies

There were three problem areas regarding territorial rights: (1) some physicians felt their authority or time was being usurped by the study staff and its activities, (2) some of the patients and medical personnel thought that the research and hospice staff were one and the same, and (3) some medical staff members attending the control group feared that they would be "shown up" by the hospice. Although these problems have not proven to be serious, they tended to persist and required the attention of the study staff on a continuing basis.

Lowered Hospice Patient Census

Randomization removes a portion of patients who are hospice-eligible from the hospice target population. Because the ratio of experimental to control patient is one to one, a hospice receives only half of those hospice-eligible patients who are both willing and able to sign an informed-consent form. Although the number of patients who refused to participate in the study or who were unable to participate is small, their number further reduces the hospice-eligible pool and thereby the number of patients who will ultimately reach the hospice. As a result, there may be momentary or steady drops in the patient census, thereby reducing the work loads for the hospice staff. As long as the number of patients who are deemed hospice-eligible exceeds the hospice's capacity to care for them, it is merely a matter of finding methods of increasing the flow from the universe of hospice-eligible patients to the hospice, keeping in mind that a portion of those assigned will go to the control group. If necessary, another technique can be used, altering the randomization ratio. Instead of having a one to one ratio, it may be possible to have a three to two ratio, whereby for every three patients who are assigned to the hospice, only two are assigned to the control group. Although such a change will reduce the size of the control group, it remains a viable way of correcting an underpopulated hospice during an experimental evaluation.

Summary and Suggestions

Despite the popularity of the hospice movement, the exact value of hospice care techniques has not been proven. To commit limited health care dollars to a new mode of treatment without the benefit of knowing its relative effectiveness and cost is unfortunate. With Congress now approving monies to reimburse patients for hospice care, the lack of scientifically sound evaluation data on hospice effectiveness is glaring.

Evaluation data can be useful for all the constituencies of the hospice — the patients and families receiving the care, the staff providing the care, administrators coordinating the care and its financing in the larger health care system, and members of the community anxious to have the hospice available to them should it be needed. The data, properly gathered, can guide administrators in determining which hospices may be ineffectual, too costly, or both, so that a decision can be reached regarding their continuation. For hospice staff, evaluation data can point the way to more effective organization and delivery of services. For the patients and their families, evaluation data assure them that hospice care is truly better and worth a wait should it be required.

Finally, for those interested in undertaking an evaluation of a hospice or a group of hospices, there are several factors to keep in mind.[34] First, an evaluation can be done within the hospice itself, by its parent organization (often the hospital of which it is a part), by an outside organization such as a university, or by private or university-affiliated consultants. Second, the size, scope, and purpose of an evaluation varies greatly, from the large, complex studies being carried out at Brown University and UCLA to very limited, week-long assessments of a topic as routine as administrative efficiency. Third, a hospice evaluation can be done once, periodically, or on a continuing basis, depending on need and available resources. Fourth, the cost can vary greatly, from nominal amounts paid for by a hospice's own budget to large amounts paid for by research grants, depending on the scope of the questions, staff requirements, supplies, and computer time.

The important point is that hospice evaluations must be done, and their results must be carefully considered if hospices are to reach their greatest potential for patients and family members, for hospice staff, and for the communities and the American society that makes them possible.

Appendix — Results of the UCLA Study

After chapter 7 was submitted for inclusion in this book, the results of the UCLA Hospice Evaluation Study were published.[35] These results are summarized here.

Terminally ill cancer patients at the Wadsworth VA Hospital in Los Angeles were randomly assigned to receive hospice or conventional care. The hospice care was provided both in a special inpatient hospice unit and at home; the conventional care was provided in the hospital, utilizing the services that are generally available to patients in that hospital. In all, 137 hospice patients and 110 control patients and their family caregivers were followed until the patient's death.

The mean age of both groups was about 64, with a range of 34 to 92. Because the study was based at a VA hospital, patients were almost all male. Most subjects were or had been employed, usually in blue-collar activities. The primary cancer sites were similarly distributed in the two groups, lung being the most common site.

The survival curves for the hospice and the control groups were essentially the same. Despite the hospice philosophy eschewing heroic efforts to extend the life of a dying patient, hospice patients died no sooner than did controls. One-third of the group died within 45 days after enrollment in the study, the second third within 120 days.

Almost 60 percent of the hospice patients who died during the study period expired in the hospice, and another third died on the general wards of the hospital; only 3 percent died at home. Of controls, almost 80 percent died in the hospital and 7 percent died at home. The rest of the deaths for both groups occurred at other institutions, usually nursing homes.

The total number of inpatient days was tabulated for both hospice patients and controls. Hospice patients spent an average of 51 days as inpatients, control patients an average of 47.5 days. There were no significant differences in the total number of days spent in the hospital by hospice and control patients.

Because hospice care attempts to improve the patient's last days by reducing or eliminating invasive diagnostic procedures and curtailing treatments such as radiation, chemotherapy, and surgery, one would expect to find fewer of these procedures among hospice patients. Analysis of the results revealed only two significant differences between hospice and control groups, for both of which hospice patients had significantly more than controls. The majority of both groups had no treatment. Of hospice patients, 74 percent had no surgery, 62 percent had no radiation, and 84 percent no chemotherapy. The corresponding figures for controls were 82 percent, 52 percent, and 84 percent. The differences in proportion were not statistically significant for any treatment category.

With regard to control of pain and other symptoms, only 41 percent of hospice patients and 38 percent of control patients reported pain at the time of entry into the study. Over the course of the study, 34 percent of hospice subjects and 31 percent of control subjects *never* reported pain. Neither of these differences was statistically significant. There was no significant difference between the groups in the proportion of subjects with pain over time. For patients experiencing pain, there were no differences in mean pain score at any time in the study.

No differences were found in the scores for other symptoms, whether all symptoms or only those most closely related to cancer were examined. No significant differences in activities-of-daily-living scores were observed between the groups. Control patients were more depressed than hospice patients, but none of the cohorts showed a statistically significant treatment effect for either depression or anxiety.

Significant differences do emerge in satisfaction scores for the hospice patients and the controls. In two of the three areas examined, hospice patients expressed more satisfaction than did control patients. For interpersonal care, all five cohort analyses that were carried out showed significant differences; for involvement in care, four of the five cohort analyses were significant.

To assess how difference in utilization of services might affect total costs, the researchers assigned prices to the various inpatient and nursing home services and then compared the hospice and control groups. The total mean inpatient cost per hospice patient was about the same as for the controls, and there were no significant differences between the hospice and control group for any of the specific categories of services.

In summary, no significant differences were noted between the hospice group and the control group in measures of pain, symptoms, activities of daily living, or affect. Hospice patients expressed more satisfaction with the care they received, and the hospice patients' family caregivers showed somewhat more satisfaction and less anxiety than did those of controls. Hospice care was not associated with a reduced use of hospital inpatient days or therapeutic procedures and was at least as expensive as conventional care.

References

1. Dupee, R. M. Hospice—compassionate, comprehensive approach to terminal care. *Postgraduate Medicine.* 1982 Sept. 72(3):234-41, 244-46.

2. Stoddard, S. *The hospice movement: A better way of caring for the dying.* New York: Stein & Day, 1978.

3. Butler, R. N. A humanistic approach to our last days. *Archives of the Foundation of Thanatology.* 1980. 8(1):59-60.

4. Saunders, C. Hospice care. *American Journal of Medicine.* 1978 Nov. 65(5):726-28.

5. Davidson, G. W. Five models for hospice care. *Quality Review Bulletin.* 1979 May. 5(5):8-9.

6. Holden, C. The hospice movement and its implications. *Annals of the American Academy of Political and Social Science.* 1980 Jan. (447):59-63.

7. Rossi, P., Freeman, H., and Wright, S. *Evaluation: A systematic approach.* Beverly Hills, CA: Sage Publications, 1979, p. 33.

8. Ames, R. P. Unresolved issues in hospice care: Models, pain control, volunteer's role. *Hospital Progress.* 1981 Mar. 45-51.

9. Buckingham, R. W., and Lupu, D. A comparative study of hospice services in the United States. *American Journal of Public Health.* 1982 May. 72(5):455-63.

10. Hinton, J. Comparison of places and policies for terminal care. *Lancet.* 1979 Jan. 6. 29-32.

11. Parkes, C. M. Terminal care: Evaluation of inpatient service at St. Christopher's Hospice. Part I: Views of surviving spouse on effects of the service on the patient. *Postgraduate Medicine.* 1979 Sept. 55:517-22.

12. Parkes, C. M. Terminal care: Evaluation of inpatient service at St. Christopher's Hospice. Part II: Self-assessments of effects of the service on surviving spouses. *Postgraduate Medicine.* 1979 Sept. 55:523-27.

13. Parkes, C. M. Terminal care: Evaluation of an advisory domiciliary service at St. Christopher's Hospice. *Postgraduate Medicine.* 1980 Oct. 56:685-89.

14. Barzelai, L. Evaluation of a home-based hospice. *Journal of Family Practice.* 1981 Feb. 12(2):241-45.

15. Silver, S. Evaluation of a hospice program: Effects on terminally ill patients and their families. *Evaluation and the Health Professions.* 1981 Sept. 4(3):306-15.

16. Van de Creek, L. A home-care hospice profile: Description, evaluation and cost analysis. *The Journal of Family Practice.* 1982. 14(1):53-58.

17. Kay, L. L., Cummings, M. A., and Mundell, M. B. Hospice: A cost analysis of three programs. Kaiser-Permanente Medical Care Program, Southern California Region. Funded by National Cancer Institute, Contract No. 85375, 1981 July.

18. Greer, D., and Mor, V. An overview of the National Hospice Study. Unpublished report, Brown University, Providence, RI, n.d.

19. Mor, V., and Birnbaum, H. Medicare legislation for hospice care: Implications of National Hospice Study data. *Health Affairs.* 1983. 2:80-90.

20. Wales, J., Kane, R., and others. UCLA hospice evaluation study: Methodology and instrumentation. *Medical Care.* 1983. 21:734-44.

21. Rossi, Freeman, and Wright.

22. Campbell, D., and Stanley, J. *Experimental and Quasi-experimental Designs for Research.* Chicago: Rand McNally, 1963.

23. Campbell and Stanley.

24. Byar, D. P., Simon, R. M., and others. Randomized clinical trials: Perspective on some recent ideas. *New England Journal of Medicine.* 1976. 195:74.

25. Wortman, P. M. Randomized clinical trials. In: Wortman, P., editor. *Methods for Evaluating Health Services.* Beverly Hills, CA: Sage Publications, 1981.

26. Melzack, R. The McGill pain questionnaire: Major properties and scoring methods. *Pain.* 1975. 1:277.

27. Ware, J. E., Snyder, M. K., and Wright, W. R. *Development and Validation of Scales to Measure Patient Satisfaction with Health Care Services.* Washington, DC: National Technical Information Service Publication No. PB28-329, 1976.

28. Selltiz, C., Wrightsman, L., and Cook, S. *Research Methods in Social Relations.* 3rd ed. New York: Holt, Rinehart, & Winston, 1976, p. 90.

29. Campbell and Stanley.

30. Campbell and Stanley.

31. Byar, Simon, and others.

32. Wortman.

33. Wales, J., Kane, R., and Krasnow, R. Using the experimental method to evaluate the impact of a hospital-based hospice program. Paper presented at the annual meeting of the Gerontological Society, Toronto, Ontario, Canada, 1981 Nov. 10.

34. For introductory reading on evaluation research in general (little is written on hospice evaluation itself), consult Rossi, P. H., and Freeman, H.E. *Evaluation: A Systematic Approach.* 2nd ed. Beverly Hills, CA: Sage Publications, 1982.

35. Kane, R., Wales, J., and others. A randomized controlled trial of hospice care. *Lancet.* 1984 April 21. 1(8382):890-94.

Chapter 8

Current Status of Hospice Financing

Mary Cummings, Dr.P.H.

Ever since their inception in the United States in the early 1970s, hospice programs have been organized and operated as relatively low-budget ventures, depending heavily on volunteered services and donations from grateful families and local foundations. Not much attention was paid to the development of accounting and billing systems, because there were no insurance mechanisms available for payment of hospice care and there was little expertise in finance among the people organizing the hospices.

Indeed, the very spirit and sense of purpose of most hospice programs made any interest in financing and reimbursement seem crass and somewhat repugnant. Most of the people joining in the early hospice efforts did so out of a sense of high idealism; their intentions were to provide a badly needed service to dying patients — to all dying patients — both those who could pay and those who could not. Considerations of costs, accounting systems, or reimbursement mechanisms simply were not given much time or energy in the development of these programs.

In recent years, however, it has become obvious that this situation is not tenable for hospice over the long run. It has become quite evident that good hospice programs require competent professional staffs, and it has also become evident that these staffs cost money — more money than has generally been available through individual donations and volunteered services. It is clear that more stable, continuous, and long-term financing mechanisms will be necessary if hospice programs are to plan appropriately for their future development. This means that hospice programs must move under the coverage of the standard health insurance plans, at least to some degree.

At the same time as these realizations have been emerging within the hospice programs themselves, parallel developments have been taking place in the health insurance system outside hospice programs. Various employers have begun to offer their employees hospice coverage as part of their standard health insurance benefits, and a number of Blue Cross and Blue Shield plans have begun to experiment with partial or full hospice coverage for their subscribers. Finally, the Congress of the United States has passed legislation to include a hospice benefit under Medicare that may benefit an estimated 274,000 terminally ill persons and their families by 1987.[1]

This chapter will discuss these developments and the issues related to the financing of hospice care in the United States. It will review studies on the cost of hospice care as well as surveys of hospice programs themselves. Present reimbursement of hospice care will be detailed, and the Medicare hospice legislation will be discussed. The chapter will close with a presentation of some of the issues for hospice financing in the future.

Preliminary Considerations

Before the question of financing hospice care is directly confronted, several preliminary issues need to be discussed. These issues run throughout all aspects of hospice financing and will affect in a major way the reader's interpretation of what is said in this chapter.

The first point to emphasize is the inadequacy of current hospice financial data for the purposes of accurate cost projections or comparisons. Although there are numerous reports related to hospice financing, they must be viewed as preliminary and descriptive in nature, not as definitive, complete, or comparable to one another.

There are several reasons for saying this. First, because there is no uniform accounting system in place to which all hospice programs subscribe, individual programs will report their financial affairs in different ways. Sometimes the same terms will be used, but the definitions will be different; other times different terms will be used to mean the same thing. For example, some programs will report costs and mean the amount it takes to operate their programs. Some programs will report costs and will exclude anything having to do with volunteered or donated services, meaning that their costs are only those items for which money must be paid out. Other programs will report costs and will include volunteered services by estimating their value or cost if they had to be purchased. Some programs will report their daily cost per patient in the hospice program, including only costs while the patient is at home and excluding whatever costs may be incurred in a hospital or an inpatient hospice. Other programs may include costs while the patient is in an inpatient hospice but not while in a hospital. Such differences make it very difficult to develop a comparable average cost per patient day. Some programs will report only on costs incurred by the hospice program itself in providing its services to patients, ignoring or omitting any additional costs incurred by the patients or families for care outside the hospice program; others will attempt to include or at least to estimate those additional costs to patients or to other health care providers.

Compounding the problem of noncomparable financial data is the fact that the hospice programs themselves are very different, not only in their forms of organization but also in the range and intensity of services offered. One hospice program may offer a type of service that another does not offer at all, or one program may offer a type of service with very great intensity and staff resources and another may offer it in an almost perfunctory fashion. One program may offer some services itself and either contract out to purchase other services or merely arrange for patients to obtain other services on their own; another program may offer all these services with its own staff. Trying to develop an average cost per patient day in these circumstances is difficult, because the array of services included in the average patient day may vary widely.

A different kind of problem arises with attempts to develop an average cost per patient day for hospice care and then to compare that cost with an average cost per patient day for hospital care; these studies usually are carried out in order to show that the average cost per patient day in hospice is much less than the average cost per day in hospital. Unfortunately, these studies frequently use noncomparable time periods, averaging hospice costs across all days from admission to death regardless of whether services were actually provided on those days and then comparing those costs with conventional hospital costs averaged across only those days when services were actually provided.

An additional problem arises from the present inability to compare accurately the populations of dying patients that are currently under care in various hospice programs. At the present time, the patient populations being served by individual hospice programs are simply described as dying patients usually with a predicted prognosis of up to six months. There are no good measures currently being used by hospice programs that would allow the detached observer to know just how sick a particular patient population really is and therefore how intense must be the services to care for that population. At present, we treat all hospice patient populations as if they were the same, although it is beginning to appear that there may be significant differences in the patient populations of different hospice programs.

Indeed, some hospice programs may actually have different admissions criteria, either implicit or explicit, that lead to the selection of certain patients on the basis of severity of disease, insurance coverage, and presence or absence of primary caregiver. As a result of these different admissions criteria, the populations being served by different hospices may vary considerably.

In some studies of hospice financing, the research design or the methods used in various reports are simply not valid or reliable, making the reported results somewhat suspect. For example, in many cases comparisons are made between the costs of care for patients dying in hospice programs and for patients dying in conventional hospitals, under the assumption that these two groups are part of the same population and that the only different feature is their participation or lack of participation in a hospice program. In fact, these two populations may be very different to begin with, quite aside from their participation or lack of participation in hospice programs, because of the presence of factors in the disease or in the patient which have predetermined the course of the illness and its care long before the option of hospice even appeared. Until these early predetermining factors are better understood, or until some kind of random assignment can be developed to remove the effect of these predetermining factors, any direct comparisons between the two populations may be completely unwarranted.

In the same fashion, a number of reports use estimating techniques for "what would have happened" or "what will happen" that are somewhat dubious. In a number of cases, for example, physicians or others are asked to estimate how many days of inpatient hospitalization were saved by hospice or how many days of inpatient hospitalization would have been used if a particular hospice program had not been present. The accuracy of this type of estimate is notoriously suspect, and yet it has not only been used, it has appeared in both a major document on hospice from the Canadian government[2] and in a major costs estimate from the U.S. Congressional Budget Office to the Congress.[3]

Finally, most of the reports and summaries related to hospice financing concentrate almost entirely on the cost and financing of the hospice care itself but do not give the total cost of a patient's illness from beginning to end. As a result, it is impossible to know the hospice program's role in the total pattern of expenditure for the illness, and, more important, it is impossible to know whether hospice changes that *total* cost of the illness at all. All of the studies that have projected hospice programs as having major cost-saving results have presumed that hospices will be used as substitutes for more traditional care, whereas skeptics have contended that hospices will be used in addition to other care, thereby increasing the total cost of care. It is inappropriate for hospice advocates to claim cost savings until better data are available about the total cost of illness.

Nonstandardized accounting and reporting systems using incomplete data, wide variability in program content and intensity, flawed research designs and estimating methods, lack of documentation of total costs of patient care per illness—all these make definitive discussion of hospice financing very difficult, and great caution should be used in drawing broad conclusions in this area. Even with all of these shortcomings, however, interesting insights are beginning to emerge and are important to note.

Nationwide Studies of Hospice Financing and Costs

Several nationwide surveys of hospice programs that include data on the costs and the financing of hospice care have been carried out. Although the results must be viewed with the caution just mentioned, they do provide a general picture of the basic financial status of hospice programs in the United States.

In 1978, the U.S. General Accounting Office was requested by senators Abraham Ribicoff, Edward Kennedy, and Robert Dole to review hospice programs in the United States in order to document many of their characteristics; included in those characteristics to be surveyed were the costs of operating the hospice programs and the sources of funding to meet those costs.[4]

Fifty-nine organizations defined themselves as hospices for the purpose of that survey, and 73 others stated that they were in the planning stages. Forty-two hospices indicated that their initial funding ranged from $100 to $3 million and came from five major sources: private donations; membership fees; hospital revenues that exceed expenses; federal, state, and local grants; contracts and private grants. Operating costs were reported as being dependent on the mix of services provided and the resulting staffing patterns. In this survey, total operating costs were reported as low as $17,202 and as high as $668,560.

In 1979, the National Hospice Organization, the Health Service Foundation (an affiliate of the Blue Cross and Blue Shield Association), and the Hospital Research and Educational Trust (an affiliate of the American Hospital Association) initiated and completed a six-month project designed to: "(1) investigate the current status of delivery systems for hospice services, identifying major issues or unmet needs, and (2) investigate the current status of payment for hospice services, again identifying major issues or unmet needs."[5] Part of their methodology was to survey 20 hospice programs that represented different models of organization, while at the same time not claiming any representativeness of the sample.

The survey found that costs for home care in the 20 programs were estimated at $33 per day and for inpatient care at $150 per day. Home care days averaged 27 days per patient, and inpatient days averaged 15 per patient. Average total cost per patient was $3,141. Interviews with 12 administrators of these hospice programs regarding the reimbursement status of hospice home care services provided the following information:

- Reimbursement to the hospices for home care services was most frequently provided by Medicare.

- Ten of the 12 programs indicated that 50 percent to 80 percent of their patients had Medicare coverage.
- Medicaid provided coverage for 2 percent to 30 percent of the patients in 8 programs.
- Blue Cross and Blue Shield covered 4 percent to 84 percent of patients in 10 programs, and commercial insurance covered 3 percent to 22 percent of patients in 8 programs.

The California State Department of Health Services conducted a one-year study of hospice care in California as authorized by Assembly Bill 1586 in 1979.[6] Four hospice programs were selected for study in different parts of the state. The purposes of the study were: (1) to determine whether Medi-Cal reimbursement should be made available for hospice care and, if so, to make recommendations on rates and regulations, (2) to assess the quality and cost-effectiveness of (a) use of lay volunteers for hospice care, and (b) hospice care versus traditional care and institutional hospice care versus in-home hospice care; and (3) to assess the current and projected demand for hospice care and the need for construction of hospice facilities and/or use of existing facilities.

For an 11-month period (1979-1980), data were collected on 252 patient-family units. The average length of stay in the hospice programs was 49 days, and about 25 percent of the patients were Medi-Cal (Medicaid) eligible. When the costs of hospice care were compared to the costs of traditional care, there appeared to be a potential for cost savings if hospice care was used, as it seemed that these hospice programs were effective in keeping patients at home longer, thus resulting in fewer acute care hospital days. It was felt that the evidence was not conclusive enough to recommend inclusion of hospice benefits in the standard Medi-Cal coverage, but recommendations were made that certain guidelines and payment policies be reviewed to determine how the existing benefits could be used to cover the more important hospice services.

Buckingham and Lupu studied 24 hospice programs that had been in operation at least one year and that had served at least 100 patients.[7] They described, among other findings, the emergence of two divergent types of hospices, those that were independent and heavily volunteer-staffed with unstable funding, and those that were institutionally based and experiencing fewer funding problems.

Some of the programs were unable to provide specific breakdowns of budget allocations and funding sources, and three programs of the 24 were not able to provide information on total annual budgets at all. Sources of funding were individual and foundation donors, third-party insurance carriers (both public and private), state and local governments, and grants from federal agencies. Five programs of the 24 reported receiving an average of $117,400 (ranging from $15,000 to $192,000) in Medicare reimbursement, and private donations ranged from $1,000 to $582,000 yearly.

Fifty-seven percent of the 24 programs surveyed reported they had experienced operating deficits in the previous fiscal year and cited lack of reimbursement for bereavement services and the need for longer-than-ordinary home care visits as reasons. The authors roughly estimated an average per-patient cost of $1,169 (with a median of $851 and a range of $64 to $3,338), limited just to the services provided by the individual hospices and not including services provided by other agencies.

The Joint Commission on Accreditation of Hospitals (JCAH) carried out a national study of hospice programs in 1981 with support from the Kellogg Foundation.[8] The major thrust of the survey was to "investigate the state of the art of hospice in the United States, to project future trends, and to estimate the impact hospice has had on other systems." The survey was primarily focused on questions related to possible accreditation of hospice programs in the future. Certain financial information was obtained from individual hospices during the course of the survey, and a special effort was made to obtain information from insurance carriers and employers as well.

A questionnaire was mailed to 800 hospices, yielding a response of 77 percent. There were 440 operational programs at the time of the survey, with most being relatively new and small. Seventy-five percent admitted fewer than 100 patient-family units in the year prior to the survey. The average monthly census was 17 patients, with an average bereavement case load of 28. Forty-six percent of the hospices were hospital-based or hospital-sponsored, 26 percent were a combination of visiting nurse associations, community-based home care agencies, or case-manager programs, 23 percent were sponsored by home health agencies, and 4 percent were totally volunteers. One hundred forty-six of the hospices (33 percent of the operational hospices) were not licensed at all, and the rest had a variety of licenses covering their operations. Sixty percent of the hospices in the JCAH survey had annual budgets under $75,000, and only 10 percent reported budgets over $300,000. Approximately half of the hospice programs surveyed reported receiving more than 40 percent of their budgets from foundations and donations.

An effort was also made in the JCAH study to contact labor unions, employers, and health insurance carriers to obtain their perspective on hospice care. Of the 177 corporations that responded to a mailed survey (35 percent), only 5 percent reported separate hospice benefits in their medical insurance policies. The majority stated that they would include hospice benefits if the programs were eventually licensed, accredited, and shown to be cost-effective. The unions surveyed responded in similar fashion to the corporations on most questions, with the exception that 13 percent reported having a hospice benefit in their medical insurance policies. Because only 13 percent of the unions surveyed responded to the survey, however, and because it is more likely that a union with a hospice benefit would respond, this figure must be viewed cautiously. The health insurance industry response to the survey (46 percent) showed a great interest in hospice programs, but only 2 percent reported an actual hospice benefit listed in their medical insurance policies at the time of the survey. The Blue Cross and Blue Shield Association reported that there were 19 pilot programs across the country, with 37 plans offering hospice benefit coverage.

In 1981 a major national study of hospice programs was begun, sponsored jointly by the Health Care Financing Administration, the Robert Wood Johnson Foundation, and the John A. Hartford Foundation.[9] In this study, 26 hospice programs were selected to receive reimbursement for hospice services provided to Medicare beneficiaries, and the experience of these hospice programs will be compared with the experiences of a group of hospices and conventional care programs not receiving special reimbursement for hospice care. The major questions in this study are as follows:

1. What is the differential impact of hospice care, whether reimbursed by Medicare or not, on the quality of life of terminally ill patients and their families, as compared to conventional or customary care?
2. What are the differential costs of caring for comparable terminally ill patients in hospices receiving special Medicare reimbursement, in hospices not receiving the special reimbursement, and in conventional care settings?
3. What is the likely impact of Medicare reimbursement on the organizational structure, staffing pattern, and costs of hospice care?
3. What will be the likely national utilization and cost of hospice care if Medicare reimbursement is extended to all authorized hospice programs and all Medicare beneficiaries?

The conclusions that can be drawn from these national studies can only be very general in nature. It seems that hospice programs are generally small with low budgets, a significant percentage of which comes from donations from individuals and grants from foundations. On the other hand, a surprising number reported that they were already receiving reimbursement from Medicare and Medicaid under existing regulations, even before any specific hospice reimbursement program went into effect. Finally, there seems to be considerable interest among labor unions and insurance carriers concerning possible hospice coverage, although there are only limited programs of coverage in place at the present time.

Financing and Cost Studies of Individual Hospices

A number of individual hospices have reported figures on the costs of providing care in their particular programs, and although the data are neither exact and complete for each program nor comparable to other programs, they are useful to review.

In a letter to the editor of the *Journal of the American Medical Association* in 1979, Sylvia Lack, M.B., the medical director at the Connecticut Hospice, indicated that the total cost for a patient and family with a mean length of stay of 10 weeks within the program was $1,200.[10] Later figures from the Connecticut hospice show a rise in cost, probably due in part to the opening of the freestanding inpatient facility as well as other factors. As of late 1982, the cost for 35 days of home care was $2,000, and the cost for a mixture of 11 inpatient days plus 38 home care days totaled $4,500. For 55 percent of the patients cared for at Connecticut Hospice, the average cost per patient was $2,000; for another 33 percent of the patients, the average cost was $6,000.[11]

The hospice program at St. Luke's Hospital Center in New York City provides care through the use of a multidisciplinary consultative team. Five types of service are offered: inpatient management, home care, clinic treatment, bereavement counseling, and single contact consultation with attending physicians. A cost analysis of approximately 300 hospice patients cared for from April 1975 through December 1979 indicated a cost of slightly more than $1,000 per case for the services of the hospice team.[12] No information is provided, however, about length of stay in the program and how much of that time was spent in the hospital and how much at home.

An outpatient hospice program has been developed at the 1,000-bed Grady Memorial Hospital in Atlanta, a hospital that services a mostly indigent population.[13] Both Joan Lipovsky, the nursing coordinator for that hospice program, and Phillip Tamson, an assistant administrator of the hospital, agree that the outpatient hospice program has reduced costs for the hospital. Seventy-five percent of the hospice patients cared for by this outpatient hospice died at home, and Tamson estimated that the hospital saved roughly $100,000 in 1980 as a result of the hospice program. This figure resulted from the savings of $333 for every day that a hospice patient was out of the hospital.

The Hospice of Columbus in Columbus, Ohio, analyzed its first year of operation as a home care hospice and reported that it cared for 70 patients during that year. These patients had an average length of stay of 42 days, at a cost of $65 per patient day.[14]

Carney and Burns are in the process of a five-year study (1980-1985) of the Community Hospice of St. Joseph in Fort Worth, Texas, a hospice that is primarily a home care program using beds in a hospital and a nursing home for inpatient care.[15,16] Preliminary results regarding the 81 patients who died during the hospice's first year of service showed that patients had an average length of stay of 36 days, an average cost per patient day of $46, and an average total cost of $1,650. The authors indicated that their average cost figures were somewhat high because they were derived from records of patients who had died; patients who were still alive and being cared for during the time of the study were not included, but if they had been, the average cost per patient being served per day would obviously be somewhat lower. The average total cost per case of $1,650 did not include cost of inpatient care in hospitals or nursing homes and was limited to costs of the hospice program itself.

Comparative Studies of Hospice Cost and Financing

In addition to the studies just mentioned, which basically reviewed the costs of providing care in only one hospice program, there have been a number of studies that not only reported on the costs of care in a particular hospice or group of hospices but also attempted to carry out some comparisons of these costs with some other form of care for terminally ill patients.

Description of Studies

A pilot study of the billed charges of terminally ill patients was carried out by Bloom and Kissick in 1980.[17] The study looked at the last two weeks of life of patients dying with malignant diseases and compared the costs of those who spent the last two weeks in a hospital with costs of those who spent the last two weeks at home and died there. Not surprisingly, the costs were 10.5 times greater for those who died in the hospital than for those who died at home. The authors suggest that this difference was due to the greater range and larger quantity of diagnostic and therapeutic services provided to the hospitalized patients. They further state that cost did not appear to be a factor in the choice of home care, as all study participants had Medicare or Blue Cross insurance coverage and were eligible for home care coverage if they had desired it. Because the patients were not randomly assigned into the two groups, it is unclear that similar populations were actually being compared. Also, the hospitals studied were university teaching hospitals, whose average costs are significantly higher even than community hospitals, further skewing the results in favor of the hospice programs.

Kassakian and Bailey reported on a clinical research study in Vermont that is reviewing the impact of home interventions made by nurse practitioners on the quality of life of advanced cancer patients.[18] In the study, a retrospective review of the last month of life for 71 patients was carried out, in order to examine a number of factors related to the cost of providing care: numbers of visiting-nurse home visits, hospital days, physician home visits, physician office visits, physician hospital visits, and nursing home costs. Several categories of patients were defined according to their place of death: "home-hospital deaths" for those who died at home, "nursing home deaths" for those who died in nursing homes, and "hospital deaths" for those who died in hospitals.

Those patients who died at home had a relative cost of care of $561. Those who died in nursing homes had a much higher relative cost, $1,496. Those who died in hospitals had the highest relative cost of all groups, $1,896. Without detailing their methodology, the authors also provide a projected relative cost of hospice care, $1,043, lower than both hospital and nursing home, but considerably higher than home nursing care provided at present. The authors concluded that although there are difficulties, patients can be cared for at home through the final stages of their terminal illness; they also concluded that there is an apparent economic benefit from such an approach and also a very real psychological benefit to both patients and families.

One of the first attempts at studying a hospice program was carried out in 1976 at the Royal Victoria Hospital, Montreal, Canada, and included an analysis of the costs of providing care.[19] Personnel salaries and laboratory tests for inpatients were assessed for a selected group of patients from the Royal Victoria Hospital hospice program (Palliative Care Unit) and a matched group of patients dying in the Royal Victoria Hospital outside that special unit. The home care program costs for hospice patients were analyzed and compared to the estimated cost of hospitalization that would have been required in the absence of this program.

The Palliative Care Unit inpatients received an average of 1.93 more hours of care per 24-hour period than did the control group of dying inpatients in other parts of the hospital. This added care led to an increased staff cost per PCU patient per day of $9.65 (at 1975-1976 salary rates). With a median hospital stay of 8.7 days, the cost of laboratory tests for PCU patients averaged $7.97; the same average cost for non-PCU patients dying in other parts of the hospital was $149.61.

Over a three-month period in 1976, home care nurses from the Palliative Care Unit made assessments at each of their home visits to determine whether the patient would have needed hospitalization if the PCU home care program did not exist. It was estimated that in the absence of the home care program, 50.5 percent of the patient days at home would have been inpatient hospital days instead; the savings per patient day was estimated at $80. Even at that early date, however, the authors recognized that true savings would not occur unless other services were discontinued; that is, the savings would only occur if the hospice services were substituted for the more expensive inpatient services, not simply added to them.

A study of the cost of providing terminal care was carried out at the hospice program of the Kaiser-Permanente Medical Center in Hayward, California, by Walter in 1979.[20] A comparative analysis was done of the costs of caring for a group of terminally ill cancer patients in the hospital before the hospice program opened, and of another group cared for in the hospice after it opened. The direct comparison of costs during the last

60 days of life showed a mean reduction in per-patient costs of $813 (17 percent), from a total cost of care of $4,424 per patient for the group treated in the hospital, to a total cost of $3,607 per patient for the group treated in the hospice. The per diem cost dropped from $266 per day for the hospital-treated group to $232 per day for the hospice-treated group. Even though the cost of nursing care in the hospice and the home was higher for the hospice group, this final cost savings resulted from a markedly lower use of ancillary services (laboratory tests and x-rays) for the hospice patients.

In 1980, a comparison study of hospice and nonhospice care was carried out in the southern California region of the Kaiser-Permanente Medical Care Program, where an inpatient hospice unit had been established some time before.[21] The time period under study was the last 28 days of life of the patient. The hospice patient sample included all patients who died in the Kaiser-Permanente hospice program at Norwalk, California. The nonhospice sample consisted of patients selected from all Kaiser-Permanente Los Angeles Medical Center patients who died during 1978 (before the Norwalk hospice opened) and who would have been eligible for hospice care had it existed at the time of their death.

The average cost per patient for nonhospice care during the last month of life was $3,562, which was 22 percent more than the cost of hospice care during the last month of life, $2,929. For both hospice and nonhospice care, over three-quarters of the per-patient costs were associated with inpatient per diem costs. The average number of inpatient days utilized during the last month of life was slightly higher in the nonhospice setting (11.44 days) than in the hospice setting (10.47 days). The small difference suggests that hospice inpatient days were almost a substitute for hospital inpatient days in the last 28 days of life. Nursing care was different in content between the two settings as well, with the hospice inpatient nurses spending substantially more time teaching patients and their families and supporting their emotional needs than did their counterparts in the standard hospital inpatient units.

In 1981, a study of the costs of providing hospice care at three freestanding hospice programs was carried out under the auspices of the National Cancer Institute.[22] The three hospices studied were the Hillhaven Hospice in Tucson, Arizona, the Kaiser-Permanente Hospice in Norwalk, California, and the Riverside Hospice in Boonton, New Jersey. The objective of the study was to compare and contrast the cost of providing the average home care visit and the average inpatient day, as well as to compare the total hospice cost per patient. Results of the study are shown in table 3, next page.

At Hillhaven Hospice, the average cost per hospice program day was $73 (mean length of stay, 43.9 days), and at the Kaiser-Permanente Hospice, the cost was $88 (mean length of stay, 51.8 days). The average cost per hospice program day per patient at the Riverside Hospice was

Table 3. Cost of Care at Three Freestanding Hospice Programs, 1979-1980

	Cost per Home Care Visit, $	Cost per Inpatient Day, $	Total Hospice Cost per Patient, $
Hillhaven Hospice	91.37	143.44	3,104.36
Kaiser-Permanente Hospice	90.94	306.50	4,554.45
Riverside Hospice	60.57	249.92	3,222.94

$57, with a mean length of stay in the program of 56.5 days. The authors of the study concluded that differences in salary levels among the three sites led to much of the cost differential, as did some variation in staffing levels. Also, because the three programs were still relatively new when studied, there were wide fluctuations in utilization of the programs, with some resulting higher costs per patient. One major advantage of this study was the fact that all costs of care except for patient-family out-of-pocket costs were included.

In 1980 Gravely and Breindel carried out a study of the costs of an inpatient hospice program at Church Hospital in Baltimore, surveying a hospice program that did not have a single concentration of inpatient beds for its patients, but that utilized beds scattered throughout the hospital as the need arose.[23] They found that the cost per admission and the cost per day for a hospice patient ($1,921 and $174, respectively) was less than that for a nonhospice medical patient ($3,431 and $345, respectively). The average length of inpatient care for hospice patients was 14.8 days (reduced to 12.1 days when the abnormally high lengths of stay of two patients were deleted from the study) as compared to nonhospice medical/surgical patients who had an average length of stay of 10.4 days. The average length of stay in the hospice program in total (inpatient and home care) was 38.1 days.

In contrast to the findings of other hospice analysts, Gravely and Breindel found that, although the length of stay of hospice patients was longer than that of nonhospice patients, the actual nursing care time was less, 3.9 hours per hospice patient per day in contrast to 4.4 hours per nonhospice patient per day. They attribute this reduced need for nursing care time for hospice patients to the vigorous use of volunteers to supplement nursing staff, with volunteers and family members spending an additional 3.5 hours per day per hospice patient on the average.

In 1979, Amado, Cronk, and Mileo reported on a hospice home care demonstration project carried out by the Genessee Regional Home Care

Association in Rochester, New York, with the support of the local Blue Cross program.[24] In this demonstration, Blue Cross agreed to provide reimbursement for skilled nursing care and ancillary services 24 hours a day, 7 days a week to dying patients in their home. The purpose of the demonstration was to test the hypothesis that provision of these fully reimbursed services to patients in their home would lower hospital utilization.

Fifty-five terminally ill patients were cared for during the period of the demonstration (April through September, 1978), receiving an average of 27 days of service at a mean per diem cost of $75.28 per day. Taken together, the 55 patients received a total of 1,576 days of care at home, of which their physicians estimated 943 days would have been spent in hospital if the home nursing care had not been available.

With the assistance of faculty at the University of Washington, Community Home Health Care, a home health agency in Seattle, evaluated the first three months of its hospice program in 1980 and compared patients who were in the agency's hospice program with other terminally ill patients receiving regular home care services.[25] Only minor differences were found in the intensity of services used by the two groups, but it was clear that hospice care required longer nursing visits, and hospice patients were more likely to use social work counseling and physical therapy. Although a rigorous cost analysis was not done, the study showed that the average hospice patient's charges during the study period totaled $493, as compared with $354 for terminally ill patients receiving regular home care.

The Visiting Nurse Association of Portland, Oregon, carried out a study of its hospice program, asking its patients' physicians whether there was a savings of hospital days as a result of the intervention of the VNA Hospice Home Care Team.[26] A sample of 120 patients was defined, and the patients' physicians were asked to estimate the number of hospital days saved as a result of the hospice home care program. The average length of stay in the hospice program for these 120 patients was 45.5 days, of which 18.3 days were hospital inpatient days. Physician estimates of additional hospital days saved was 7 to 14 days per patient; the cost savings per patient was estimated at $2,559.

In 1982, Group Hospitalization, Inc. (GHI), the Blue Cross plan for metropolitan Washington, DC, reported on the results of a three-year, seven-month hospice pilot project.[27] The average length of stay on the project for all GHI patients was 25.5 days, with an average per case charge of $2,343 and an average per diem charge of $92.04. For those GHI patients who used only home care services, the average length of stay was 23.2 days, the average per case charge was $2,231, and the average per diem charge was $96.18. For those GHI patients who used both hospice home care and acute care inpatient services, the average home care stay was 31.2 days and the average inpatient hospital stay was 8.8 days; the average charge per case was $5,059 with an average per diem, including both inpatient and home care, of $126.05 per day.

The difference of $2,826 in the per case cost between the two groups (home care only, and home care and inpatient care) represented to GHI a potential cost savings of $186,543, just for the patients taking part in the hospice pilot project. When the experience of all the hospice pilot project patients was compared to the average per patient cost for a terminal cancer admission to an inpatient facility without hospice services ($7,047), it was felt that the total hospice pilot project generated potential cost savings of $343,988 for GHI.[28]

In 1984, Brooks and Smyth-Staruch reviewed the experience of Blue Cross of Northeast Ohio to determine whether the addition of a hospice benefit led to substantial cost savings to the third-party insurers.[29] Their study compared the third-party payments for Cuyahoga County (Ohio) residents who died of cancer and were served by a hospice home care program (152 patients) with the insurance payments of cancer patients who never received hospice home care (1,397 patients).

A general comparison of the medical use and third-party expenditures of hospice and nonhospice cancer patients during the last 24 weeks of life did not show much cost savings for hospice home care. The hospice study subjects averaged only 1.6 fewer hospital days and 4.1 fewer nursing home days than the nonhospice patients; this difference produced a lower cost difference of $250 per patient. However, the hospice patients also averaged 12.3 more home care visits, which cost third parties an additional $507 per patient. Overall, the total bill for the entire 24-week period was slightly higher for the hospice patients ($9,651) than it was for the nonhospice patients ($9,362).

When the authors focused more carefully on time periods that were actually closer to the time of death, however, they found significant reductions in hospital use and significant relative cost savings *for those periods of time* for patients who used hospice home care services, that is, 39 percent relative savings during the last 12 weeks, 44 percent during the last 8 weeks, 47 percent during the last 4 weeks, and 51 percent during the last 2 weeks.

In 1984, Kane, Wales, and others conducted a randomized trial of hospice care in a large Veterans Administration hospital in Los Angeles. Although they did not report specific financial findings, they did show that hospice inpatient care in this setting was not associated with reduced use of hospital inpatient days or therapeutic procedures and was at least as expensive as conventional care.[30]

The most complete and detailed data about the costs of hospice care come from the National Hospice Study, preliminary reports of which are beginning to appear in reports and journals.[31,32] This study was jointly sponsored by the Health Care Financing Administration, the Robert Wood Johnson Foundation, and the John A. Hartford Foundation and was specifically designed to answer questions about the cost of hospice care and its potential for reducing costs.[33,34] It has already provided some important information about hospices and their patients, as well as about the impact of hospices on patients' condition, [35,36] and is now beginning to provide some important financial data as well.[37]

Included in the National Hospice Study were 11 hospital-based hospice programs and 14 home care hospices as the demonstration sites, along with 14 other hospices and 12 conventional care programs as nondemonstration sites or controls. Within the 25 demonstration sites, the study concentrated on Medicare patients (whose care in demonstration sites was being financed by Medicare); these included 2,746 patients in home care hospices and 1,143 patients in hospital-based hospices.

What is the cost of hospice care? The National Hospice Study suggests that a hospital-based hospice costs Medicare $95 per day and a home care hospice, $66, a difference of 44 percent between the two. Because patients in home care hospices stay in hospice longer than do hospital-based hospice patients (72.5 days for home care hospices versus 62.3 days for hospital-based hospices), the total cost per hospice admission is slightly less marked between the two types of hospice care, but still quite significant: the total cost per patient for the entire hospice admission was $5,890 for hospital-based hospices and $4,758 for home care hospices, a difference of 24 percent between the two.

Within the individual hospices, there was considerable variation among patients, with 17.9 percent of home care hospice patients and 9.4 percent of hospital-based hospice patients having total costs during the entire admission of $500 or less. At the same time, 22.8 percent of home care hospice patients and 29.3 percent of hospital-based hospice patients had total costs of $6,500 or more.

Considerable variation existed among the hospices themselves, with the average cost ranging from $30 per day in the lowest cost home care hospice to $153 per day in the highest cost hospital-based hospice. The total cost per entire hospice stay for these two hospice programs ranged from a low of $2,301 per stay for the lowest cost home care hospice to $8,595 for the highest cost hospital-based hospice.

In general, the hospital-based hospices had considerably higher costs per day and also per stay in hospice, but the results here were mixed as well. Five of the home care hospices actually had total costs that were higher than the lowest cost hospital-based hospice, and 10 of the 11 hospital-based hospices had costs that were lower than at least one (and sometimes many) home care hospices.

How can this significant variation in costs between one type of hospice and another be explained? The researchers conducting the National Hospice Study suggest that hospice costs reflect the range of services offered by a hospice, the actual level of utilization of those services, and the cost per unit of providing that service — all of which vary widely among hospices of all kinds. The cost also varies widely according to the types of patients being served and some of the important characteristics of those patients, such as category of cancer, severity of the illness and the stage at which the patient enters the program, and the availability of hospice services in the community and supportive help within the home.

When asked what the impact of hospice is on the costs of terminal care, the National Hospice Study researchers report that the results are mixed. "Whether hospice saves money depends crucially on the type of hospice and the timing in which patients enter hospice. There is no simple, unambiguous answer as to the cost or savings of hospice care. While home care hospice always seems to lead to savings, hospital-based hospice care can lead to cost increases for patients with long hospice stays (longer than two months)."[38]

Conclusions

What conclusions can be drawn from this welter of confusing and sometimes contradictory data about the costs and the financing of hospice care? What general summaries can be drawn and what implications identified from reviewing the increasing number of reports that deal with these matters? Two general areas appear to deserve comment, the first related to the actual costs of hospice care.

First, although it has been very difficult to develop standard costs for hospice care as a whole and for its component parts, much has been learned about the financing of hospice care and about the financial systems in hospices themselves.

From a financial point of view, a wide diversity exists among hospice programs, which directly reflects the wide diversity in other aspects of these programs. Their budgets range from the very small (in the tens of thousands of dollars) to the somewhat large (in the hundreds of thousands of dollars), with the average being generally on the small side (one hundred thousand dollars or less).

At the same time, virtually all programs report a steady growth in the size of their budgets, related both to the growth of the programs themselves and to their increasing ability to obtain financial support from one source or another. Their systems of accounting and financial management are still rather rudimentary, but they do show signs of increasing sophistication.

Although it is true that hospice programs in the past depended entirely on donations, grants, and volunteered services for their financial support, there is strong evidence of increasing dependence on Medicare, Medicaid, and private insurance carriers for basic financial support, even without some implementation of the Medicare hospice benefits and even without some insurance companies having formal hospice benefits in their present policies.

No definitive conclusions can be given about the actual costs of hospice care, either in total or for its individual parts, because the present data are simply inadequate for any accurate appraisal or for cross-program comparisons. Ranges for individual items of hospice care and for total hospice admissions are listed in table 4, next page, but these figures should not be used for anything more than general observations.

The second general point to be made about the costs and financing of hospice care is that it is unclear that hospice care necessarily and always is cheaper than conventional care or that hospice care always saves money for patients, insurers, and society. Evidence *is* growing that when used properly, hospice care does provide a lower cost alternative to more expensive patterns of traditional care, but the methods of decision about when and how to use hospice programs and the cost implications of these decisions are still unclear. There is no evidence that merely including hospice programs in a total pattern of care for terminally ill patients automatically and necessarily reduces the total cost of illness, although there seems to be little doubt that for some patients in some circumstances at some point in their illness, hospices do save money. The challenge now seems to be to identify more exactly those patients and those circumstances in which hospice programs are more appropriate and economical than conventional care.

Insurance Reimbursement for Hospice Care

While many developments have been taking place within hospice programs across the country, what has been the reaction of the nation's health insurance plans? How much coverage and what kind of hospice benefits are being offered now and what form are future developments likely to take?

In 1978, Cohen surveyed insurance companies in an attempt to determine what hospice benefits they offered at the time.[39] For this survey, 582 questionnnaires were mailed out, yielding a response of 145 (25 percent). Of the respondents, only 17 percent provided any hospice benefits at the time of the survey, and these were limited to traditional nursing and medical care; family counseling and bereavement services were not covered at all.

In 1981, the Frank B. Hall Company, an insurance consulting firm, conducted a survey of 11 major insurance carriers to determine what types of hospice coverage they were offering and found relatively little formal hospice coverage in effect at the time. When the study was repeated in 1982, however, a number of very significant changes were noted.[40]

The study found that by 1982, carriers had begun reimbursing hospices for care, even in the absence of specific hospice benefits, using provisions of the insurance contracts that already existed. "It is evident," said the study report, "that carriers universally embrace a moral and social responsibility to provide appropriate care for dying patients and their families. This commitment alone does not account for the dramatic shift in cover-

**Table 4. Reported Lengths of Stay and
Costs for U.S. Hospice Programs,
1979-1983**

	Length of Stay, Range in Days	Cost, Range in $
Entire stay in program	25.5 to 70.0	1,169 to 5,059
Inpatient care in program	8.6 to 18.6	143 to 306
Hospice care in program	—	33 to 96

age for hospice care by commercial insurers. It is apparent that real competitive pressure exists among carriers to evaluate and consider for inclusion cost-effective alternatives to acute care for terminally ill patients." Because of the major developments discovered in the study, it is useful to review the findings in more detail.

Blue Cross and Blue Shield

In November 1978, the national Blue Cross and Blue Shield Associations issued a joint statement regarding hospice care and payment for services. The statement expressed both support for the hospice concept and caution with regard to the financing implications.[41] This statement has generally served as the guideline for most of the developments in the individual Blue Cross and Blue Shield plans ever since.

At the time of the Hall study, more than 35 Blue Cross and Blue Shield plans offered coverage for hospice services. These services were primarily available as an extension of already existing home health care benefits, but eight plans had begun to offer specific criteria available to judge providers. Because there were no official accreditation criteria available to judge providers, most plans used their own discretion in identifying providers who would be eligible for reimbursement. The benefits offered varied widely from plan to plan, usually depending on local service availability and other local conditions, but all stressed home care and other methods of avoiding inpatient care. Counseling and bereavement services were generally not covered, unless special arrangements had been made with individual providers.

Several of the individual Blue Cross and Blue Shield pilot projects were particularly innovative and worthy of special notice. In 1978, Connecticut Blue Cross and Blue Shield made the first agreement with Connecticut Hospice to provide coverage for terminal patients treated at home. In 1980, Connecticut Blue Cross and Blue Shield became the first private insurance carrier to provide inpatient coverage at Connecticut Hospice, when that program opened its inpatient unit. The agreement covered inpatient stays of up to 60 days at a daily charge of $215 per day. Social services, bereavement counseling, and pastoral care were also covered, in addition to medical care services. As a result of providing hospice coverage, Blue Cross and Blue Shield became a major factor in the financing of Connecticut Hospice, providing 16 percent of all third-party payments of the hospice; Medicare provided the much greater share (69.6 percent), all other private insurance carriers paid 12 percent, and Medicaid paid 2.4 percent. It is instructive to note that much of the development in Connecticut was the result of a state requirement that all newly issued health insurance policies include hospice coverage.

Blue Cross and Blue Shield of Maryland instituted a pilot hospice project in 1979, with six hospital-based home care programs and one freestanding home care agency.[42] During its first two and one-half years, the home care programs served 192 patients with an average length of stay in the program of 35.4 days and an average cost per case for home care of $1,415. Inpatient hospice care had an average length of stay of 11.9 days and an average cost per case of $2,669 — both reimbursed completely by the insurance carrier.

In the Rochester, New York, area, the Blue Cross plan entered into an agreement with the Genessee Regional Home Care Association to provide reimbursement for skilled nursing and ancillary home health care 24 hours a day, 7 days a week to support dying patients.[43]

Group Hospitalization, Inc., the Blue Cross plan for the Washington, DC, area, instituted a pilot project to provide reimbursement for hospice home care services that lasted more than three years.[44] An analysis of the results indicated that the hospice pilot project generated potential cost savings of $343,988 for GHI patients, and by helping make services available in the community to both GHI and non-GHI patients, the project generated a potential cost savings of $1,047,571 for the entire area.

In late 1981, the national Blue Cross and Blue Shield Associations reviewed the hospice reimbursement experience up to that point and stated that a clear picture of hospice utilization or cost had not emerged yet because the majority of plan programs had been operational for a relatively short period of time. Early indications were that utilization had been fairly low, but it was not known whether that was due to the relative newness of the hospice programs themselves, the relative newness of the Blue Cross coverage for their services, or to other factors.

Aetna Life Insurance Company

Aetna did not have a separate hospice benefit, but it would reimburse for certain hospice services under the hospital or home health care provision of a contract, at the suggestion of the client holding that contract. For those large policyholders who requested the additional coverages, "caps" (that is, upper limits on total expenditure) were placed on those services, ranging from $3,000 to $10,000. The benefit as structured, included reimbursement for inpatient hospice care as long as that hospice program was affiliated with a licensed institution of one kind or another. The services of nurses and home health care aides were reimbursed when these providers were part of a licensed home health care agency or a visiting nurse service; the treatment plan in these home care agencies had to be coordinated by a nurse. Financial planning and bereavement counseling after the patient's death were excluded from reimbursement without a specific increase to cover these services, ranging from $0.28 to $0.88 per covered employee per month.

Aetna had a number of concerns related to insurance for hospice services. There was considerable uncertainty regarding utilization and therefore the ultimate cost of bereavement counseling. Aetna was also concerned that third-party reimbursement of hospice services would encourage the substitution of paid services for services that were previously provided by volunteers. Such a substitution would drive up the overall cost of hospice care and negate previously estimated cost savings.

Connecticut General

Connecticut General was one of the first carriers to provide hospice coverage, beginning in Connecticut in 1978. On policyholder request, hospice services were reimbursed under Connecticut General's standard comprehensive or major medical policies. Outpatient charges were reimbursed if the plan included home health care benefits, and inpatient expenses were reimbursed only if the hospice facility was part of a hospital and its services could be distinguished from those provided in a hospital.

In compliance with Connecticut law regarding contract readability, Connecticut General expanded the social services provision in its home health care benefit to include hospice services. This service included assessment of the social, psychological, and family problems related to an illness and its treatment, specifically the treatment of terminally ill patients, as mandated by law. It also covered the appropriate action taken and the use of community resources to resolve these related problems. No distinction was made between inpatient and outpatient services with regard to this social service benefit; there was a $200 limit on this provision, regardless of site of provision.

Since October 1982, Connecticut General has made progress toward the development of a separate hospice benefit. The product specifications have been drafted, and the final approval and marketing of this benefit were to begin sometime in the first half of 1983. The proposed specifications include reimbursement of inpatient and outpatient hospice services and include palliative treatment and family counseling for a specific time not yet determined. A lifetime maximum has also been proposed, but the exact amount has not yet been agreed upon. Maximum benefits and acceptable numbers of visits for bereavement counseling will be up to the individual policyholders to determine. It is expected that the cost of adding this optional hospice benefit will be minimal.

Connecticut General has not yet been convinced of the cost savings potential of establishing a hospice benefit. In its own survey, Connecticut General found that freestanding hospices did not appear to offer any cost savings potential over hospital care but that home-based hospice care did seem to have that potential. As with other carriers, Connecticut General was concerned about the lack of accreditation and quality standards. As a result, all hospices covered by its benefit were subject to review and approval by Connecticut General before reimbursement was extended for services provided in those hospices.

Equitable Life Assurance Society

Equitable offered a coordinated program of benefits with a full range of service for hospice care. The standard benefit structure provided first-dollar, full-dollar reimbursement within a $2,500 maximum for hospice expenses. When that maximum was reached, some expenses might still be covered under other parts of a client's benefit program. In addition, optional benefits allowed for a $5,000 maximum with a $50 or $100 deductible and 80 percent or 90 percent coinsurance.

The benefit period for hospice service was six months following the date of certification of terminal illness. If the benefit period ended before the death of a terminally ill patient, a new benefit period might begin if the attending physician certified that the patient was still terminally ill. The benefit period for bereavement counseling was 12 months following the death of the patient; there was a $25 allowance per bereavement session with a maximum of 12 sessions over the 12-month period.

Like Connecticut General, Equitable had established its own criteria for determining whether a hospice was qualified for reimbursement. These criteria included the requirement that the hospice program be organized and licensed as such by the state in which it was located. If accreditation was available, the program must also be currently accredited. In the event that state laws or regulations did not exist, the hospice program must be accredited by some national accrediting body or must be recognized as a demonstration hospice program by the U.S. Department of Health and Human Services or must satisfy Equitable that the program conformed to the standards required by New York state.

Equitable reported that there had not been a large volume of requests for hospice benefits during the year prior to the study and that most of the interest had been expressed by large policyholders. In line with this general experience, Equitable did not levy an additional premium for hospice coverage to policyholders with 500 or more covered employees.

Hartford Life and Accident Company

At the time of the 1982 Hall study, Hartford did not offer a hospice benefit, but it was giving serious consideration to providing such coverage in the future. Hartford indicated that there may be cost savings associated with the institution of hospice benefits, but it was unclear as to how these benefits should be structured and integrated into the rest of coverage to achieve the maximum cost savings effect.

Metropolitan Life Insurance Company

At the time of the 1982 Hall study, Metropolitan did not offer a specific hospice benefit to its policyholders, but it was planning to introduce a supplemental hospice package to those policyholders who might wish such coverage. Because of the lack of official accreditation, Metropolitan's medical department was developing its own criteria for hospice eligiblility for reimbursement. The proposed supplemental hospice benefit would focus primarily on outpatient services such as home care. Social services billed through a licensed social service agency would be eligible for reimbursement; bereavement counseling services would be considered as an option, with limits on this option yet to be determined. Metropolitan indicated that there may be some cost savings involved with the addition of a hospice benefit, but no statistics had yet fully demonstrated this fact to the company's satisfaction. When the benefit is offered to policyholders, there will be no additional premium or charge.

Mutual of Omaha Insurance Company

Mutual of Omaha does not offer a specific hospice benefit to its general policyholders, but hospice coverage could be obtained under the company's Cancer Cost Supplement. The benefit paid $30 per day for up to 100 days; after a 30-day period without treatment, another benefit period began. The annual cost for the supplemental cancer coverage package was $96 for an adult under age 59, $144 for a family with adults under age 59, $306 for an adult 60 years of age and older, and $519 for a family with an adult 60 years of age and older. Mutual of Omaha also offered hospice coverage on a group-by-group basis for those policyholders who requested it or for those policyholders who, according to state law, must be provided such a hospice benefit. A hospice benefit written for an individual group was usually included as an extension of the policyholder's home health care provision, but this did not preclude the payment for hospice services delivered in a hospital or inpatient setting. In these special group policies, Mutual of Omaha did not reimburse for bereavement counseling. At the time, there were no costs associated with adding hospice coverage.

New England Life Insurance Company

New England Life did not provide hospice coverage except in those states where it was required by state law. In those cases, the hospice services were placed under major medical provisions, where unlimited coverage was usually available for such services as home health nursing when prescribed by a physician; other services were covered under the home health care or extended medical benefits. An added premium was associated with this coverage in those states where the coverage was required by law.

New York Life Insurance Company

New York Life was developing plans to introduce hospice coverage in early 1983 as part of its major medical policies; there would be no extra charge for this coverage. The coverage would include components for both inpatient and outpatient hospice programs and would also include coverage for services of physicians, nurses, psychologists, social workers, and bereavement counselors. The services of volunteers would not be reimbursed. In the absence of formal accreditation standards, New York Life would reimburse only those hospices that met the National Hospice Organization guidelines and had the approval of New York Life.

Prudential Insurance Company of America

Prudential had developed a standard hospice benefit that was currently being marketed as a supplemental benefit to its basic medical and hospital insurance plans. The supplemental coverage included reimbursement for both inpatient and outpatient care, with a maximum outpatient benefit set at $2,000 and a maximum inpatient at $3,000 with a daily cap of $150. Bereavement counseling services were available to members of the family unit for up to $200 during the three months following the death of the patient. Prudential reimbursed for the services of a hospice team, which it defined to include at least a doctor, a registered nurse, a social worker, a clergyman/counselor, volunteers, a clinical psychologist, a physiotherapist, and an occupational therapist. To be eligible for reimbursement, each hospice care recipient must have a life expectancy certified to be six months or less.

The major reservation that Prudential had in reimbursing hospices was the lack of central licensing or accreditation standards and a body to govern these standards. In the absence of national standards, Prudential had elected to reimburse the services provided by hospices affiliated with the National Hospice Organization, which were physician-directed, nurse-coordinated, and centrally administered.

Travelers Insurance Company

Travelers currently was marketing a hospice benefit as part of a total package that was directed to all new small group policyholders. The benefits covered inpatient and outpatient services, with no limit on the number of home health services and with no requirement of prior hospital confinement in order to become eligible to receive hospice services. Bereavement counseling services were reimbursed at 50 percent, with a 15-visit limit for family members within six months after the patient's death. Covered expenses did not include services of a social worker (other than a clinical social worker) unless provided as part of the inpatient hospice program, nor did they include services provided by volunteers or individuals who did not regularly charge for their services. Hospice care services by a licensed pastoral counselor to a member of his or her congregation was not reimbursed.

Travelers had made the hospice care benefit available to small group policyholders because it was a useful marketing tool. However, because Travelers usually bid on policy specifications that were spelled out in advance by potential large group policyholders, there was no standard approach to offering hospice benefits to large groups. The large groups specified in advance what they wanted to include in the package of benefits, and if hospice care was desired, Travelers would include this as a covered benefit. At the time of the Hall study, only a few large groups had specifically requested the hospice coverage.

Travelers had not found documented evidence of cost savings by means of a hospice care benefit. There appeared to be a disparity in the actual cost savings attributed to the different hospice models, with the home care programs probably contributing considerably greater cost savings than the inpatient models. Travelers has expressed a concern that the quality of care provided by hospices might be compromised by a broad extension of health insurance coverage, which might attract self-seeking entrepreneurs who were interested only in the reimbursement and not necessarily in the personal quality of care.

Business Health Insurance Packages

In addition to the formal coverage being extended in one fashion or another by the health insurance carriers, a number of large businesses have begun to include some form of hospice benefit in the health insurance packages that they offer to their workers. General Electric, Westinghouse, and the United Auto Workers have all negotiated with various Blue Cross and Blue Shield plans for hospice benefits for their employees or members. Of the 750,000 eligible workers at General Electric, only seven had used the benefit in the first 10 months of the coverage. General Motors and Ford have been looking into the possibility of hospice care for their employees, as have TRW and several large West Coast companies.

Summary

In summary, several points can be made about the present status of insurance reimbursement for hospice services and about future directions in this area. First, it is clear that health insurance plans that are at present in effect are already being used to pay for some hospice services, even without the existence of specifically designated hospice benefits. In general, the reimbursement here is for inpatient services or for home health care services that would be covered even without their provision by a hospice program.

Second, the health insurance industry is watching the development of hospice programs closely and is generally moving toward the creation of specific hospice benefits, either as added benefits to already existing plans or as new supplemental coverage to be offered separately. The industry seems to believe that this coverage can be offered cheaply, and in some cases where the coverage is already being offered, no additional premium is being charged. Although not many data are available yet to determine utilization, there seems to be a belief that there will be relatively light utilization of this benefit, compared to the utilization of the more traditional physician and hospital coverage.

Third, the health insurance industry as a whole seems somewhat skeptical of the claims for cost savings that have been made for hospice services, even though the potential is recognized for reducing inpatient care if hospice home care benefits are utilized properly. In general, the health insurance companies that are thinking about offering hospice benefits are not doing so as part of their health care cost reduction efforts but rather as part of their more general marketing effort; they want to be seen as adding new benefits and new services as appropriate, keeping a competitive position with regard to other companies in the field.

Finally, most of the health insurance companies surveyed in the Hall study expressed concern about various aspects of expanded insurance coverage for hospice care. Chief among their concerns was the lack of a national accreditation for hospice programs that might help insurance companies know better which programs to reimburse and which to avoid. The companies are also concerned that expanded coverage might stimulate replacement of volunteer services with paid staff services, thereby having the dual negative effect of removing volunteer involvement as a significant part of hospice care and at the same time driving up costs. Finally, the insurance companies are concerned that the availability of expanded insurance coverage will attract providers who are primarily interested in taking advantage of the financial potential and who are not deeply committed to the high ideals of service that have motivated the field up to this point.

Hospice Coverage under Medicare

Status

Since November 1, 1983, terminally ill patients over 65 years of age have been eligible under Medicare for certain hospice services they receive primarily at home. The enabling legislation, which is part of the Tax Equity and Fiscal Responsibility Act passed by Congress in August 1982, represents a significant development in the history of hospice programs in the United States.[45]

Hospices have been interested in having some expanded form of coverage under Medicare for some time, because approximately 60 percent of hospice patients are over the age of 65. Although Medicare is already paying for a significant portion of the care provided by hospices (for example, 70 percent of the insurance reimbursement received by the Connecticut Hospice in 1980), it has long been felt that the development of a specific hospice benefit under Medicare would allow for a number of important services that are not now covered.

At the same time, Medicare has been concerned about the rising cost of terminal care for its recipients. For example, it is estimated that Medicare will spend almost $50 billion in 1982, accounting for one out of every $15 spent by the federal government for all purposes. Sixty-five percent of those who died in 1976 were Medicare beneficiaries, and although they represented only 6.4 percent of Medicare enrollees, they accounted for 31 percent of all Medicare payments that year.[46] Obviously, if hospice services offer the potential of cost savings to Medicare, it becomes extremely important to develop a hospice benefit that would allow for better use of these services.

In December 1981, the National Hospice Education Project, composed of a number of hospice leaders who were convinced that Medicare coverage was essential to the future of hospice, developed draft legislation that would make hospice care a benefit under Medicare. At the same time, the Warner Lambert Foundation sponsored a study by a Washington, DC, consulting firm that showed that the cost of one day of hospice care was only 20 to 25 percent of the daily cost of hospital care. The study suggested that hospice care might possibly produce net savings to Medicare of $13 million to $50 million in the first year of coverage and perhaps as much as $30 million to $150 million in the fifth year, depending on how the benefit was structured and how it was used.[47]

In early 1982, legislation was introduced by Congressman Leon Panetta of California and Senator Robert Dole of Kansas (H.R. 5180 and S. 1958) that would permit reimbursement of hospice care for patients with a life expectancy of six months or less.[48] More than 190 members of the House of Representatives joined in cosponsoring Panetta's bill in the House, and more than 28 senators served as cosponsors for Dole's proposal in the Senate.

Despite the appeal of the legislation from many points of view, caution was advised by many powerful forces, including the American Hospital Association, the national Blue Cross and Blue Shield Association, and the Reagan Administration itself. In testimony before the health subcommittee of the House Ways and Means Committee in March 1982, Paul Willging, deputy administrator of the Health Care Financing Administration, stressed that his objections were not to the concept of hospice, which he praised very strongly, but arose out of a fear of the financial consequences of the bill. He pointed out that the End-State Renal Disease Program had started out with a very limited scope and had blossomed into an incredibly expensive program, and he was concerned that the same thing might happen to the hospice benefits unless they were very carefully implemented. He urged Congress to wait until the results of the HCFA-Robert Wood Johnson-John Hartford Foundation research project was completed before final action was taken on the Panetta legislation.[49]

Neil Hollander, vice-president of the national Blue Cross and Blue Shield Association, testified in the same vein, reiterating cautions to the federal government that he had put forward several years earlier to the Blue Cross plans and to the commercial insurance carriers.[50] He pointed out that the suggested cost savings that had been discussed so frequently in the preliminary maneuverings for the Panetta legislation would only be possible if hospice was used as a substitute for expensive inpatient care, not as an addition, and the proposed legislation did not deal adequately with that problem.[51]

For a short while, until June 28, 1982, when the Congressional Budget Office provided its estimate of the impact of the legislation, it seemed as if the chances for successful passage of the Panetta-Dole legislation were doubtful.[52] Usually rather cautious and conservative in its appraisal, the CBO had a generally good reputation with legislators, so that when it estimated a net savings in 1983 of $1,120 per hospice user, the legislative issue was no longer in doubt. On August 19, 1982, the hospice bill was passed by both the House of Representatives and the Senate and was included as Section 122 of the Tax Equity and Fiscal Responsibility Act of 1982 by action of Senator John Heinz of Pennsylvania.[53]

Under the terms of the legislation, after November 1, 1983, terminally ill patients over the age of 65 and with less than six months to live would be able to use their Medicare benefits to obtain hospice services from bona fide programs of care. These eligible programs would be ones that could provide hospice care and services as needed, whether inpatient, outpatient, or home care, on a 24 hours per day, seven days per week basis. They would employ an interdisciplinary team consisting at least of one physician, one registered nurse, one social worker, and one other counselor, either psychological or pastoral. A written plan for furnishing hospice care to each individual must be established before care is provided and must be periodically reviewed by the patient's attending physician, the hospice medical director, and the interdisciplinary team. The approved hospice programs must utilize volunteer services, must be centrally organized and administered, must maintain centralized records on all patients, and must be licensed according to the prevailing laws in the state in which they provide care.

The actual package of services to be covered by the Medicare hospice legislation would include nursing care; physical and occupational therapy; speech therapy; medical social services; home health care by a trained aide; homemaker services; medical supplies, including drugs, biologicals, and appliances; physician's services; short-term inpatient care, including respite care for the family; and counseling, including bereavement counseling and dietary-nutritional counseling.

To be eligible for the hospice benefit, an individual must be certified as terminally ill within two days of initiating hospice care, such certification being carried out both by the patient's attending physician and either the hospice medical director or physician member of the hospice team. When a patient elects to use the hospice care benefit, he or she relinquishes Medicare reimbursement during the benefit period for any other services related to the terminal illness except the services of the attending physician. Should the patient decide to return to more traditional treatment service, this action will automatically bring to an end the patient's eligibility for hospice care during that benefit period.

The hospice benefit periods are divided into two 90-day periods and one 30-day period. The patient must be certified as being terminally ill to begin the first 90-day period of benefits and must be recertified as terminally ill for the following 90-day and 30-day period. The legislation also insists that over a 12-month period, a hospice program's patients not spend more than 20 percent of the aggregate number of covered days in an inpatient facility; put another way, the legislation mandates that at least 80 percent of patients' time over the 12-month period be spent at home.

With regard to total payments per patient for hospice care, the legislation sets a cap or upper limit on the total amount of money that can be paid for the care of any one hospice patient. This cap was originally set at 75 percent of the regional average per capita payments that Medicare was making for terminally ill cancer patients; that is, if the average total Medicare payment for care of terminally ill patients in traditional settings was $1,000, the ceiling amount that would be paid for all hospice services would be 75 percent, or $750. In the negotiations leading to the eventual passage of the Panetta-Dole proposal, this figure was reduced to 40 percent of the regional average of total Medicare per capita payments for terminally ill cancer patients.

Following the passage of the bill, a serious difference of opinion arose between the Congressional sponsors of the hospice Medicare legislation and the Reagan Administration officials in the Health Care Financing Administration and the Office of Management and Budget, particularly David Stockman of OMB. In their original estimates, the Congressional sponsors had assumed that the average costs for Medicare services for a terminally ill patient in the last six months of life were approximately $19,000, which would have led to a maximum hospice payment limit of between $7,000 and $8,000. However, HCFA officials estimated that the costs were actually about $11,000 in the last six months of life, leading to a maximum hospice Medicare limit of $4,200.

Virtually all the hospice leaders who had supported the original legislation were unanimous in the feeling that this "cap," or limit, on Medicare payment to a hospice was so low as to make the legislation meaningless. No hospice, it was felt, could afford to take on the care of a patient and try to fulfill the other conditions of the legislation, if the total reimbursement cap for that care was $4,200. It simply could not be done for that amount, and it was believed that most hospices would not even try to participate in the Medicare hospice benefit, because it would force them to assume responsibility for providing a range of services that the reimbursement level simply could not support.

Months of discussion followed among hospice leaders, Congressional supporters, and officials of the Health Care Financing Administration and the Office of Management and Budget, with each side standing firmly by what it felt the upper limit of the reimbursement should be. Finally, on July 27, 1983, Congressman Leon Panetta (D-Calif) and Willis Gradison (R-Ohio) introduced H.R. 3677, a bill that would set the upper limit on Medicare hospice payments at $6,500, instead of equating it to 40 percent of the costs of care during the last six months of life for cancer patients. The bill also made provisions for increasing this amount annually by an amount equal to the increase in the medical expenditure category of the Consumer Price Index. The House Ways and Means Committee approved the bill the next day, and the entire House passed it four days later on August first. The Senate, under the leadership of Finance Committee Chairman Robert Dole (R-Kans), acted on it two days later on August 3, and it was signed by the President on August 29, 1983.

The original hospice legislation also required that prior to September 30, 1983, the U.S. Department of Health and Human Services report to Congress concerning the results of the current HCFA-Robert Wood Johnson-John A. Hartford Foundation research project, the cost-effectiveness of hospice care, and the reasonableness of the 40 percent upper limit on total reimbursement. The new legislation removes the requirement to report on the upper 40 percent limitation and merely substitutes the $6,500 figure. The original legislation also required that prior to January 1, 1986, HHS report on the fairness, equitability, and efficiency of the proposed reimbursement method and benefit structure, the feasibility of moving into a system of prospective reimbursement for hospice care, and an evaluation of the methods of payment for outpatient drugs and counseling services.

Following the passage of the new amending legislation, the debate shifted to details of implementation of specific aspects of the legislation, particularly reimbursement for specific items of service and certification of eligibility of providers to take part in the Medicare benefit.

On August 22, 1983, a Notice of Proposed Rule-Making was circulated by the Health Care Financing Administration for comments, and more than 200 separate responses were received.[54] Many of the comments were used to modify the proposed rules, and on December 16, 1983, final Medicare hospice regulations were published in the *Federal Register.*[55] Specifically, the reimbursement rates for certain services that had originally been proposed in August were now modified (see table 5, next page).

A number of organizations objected to the new proposed rates, but in view of the fact that the revisions were based, at least in part, on preliminary data from the Brown University study, the new rates were generally accepted as appropriate.

A more vigorous debate has centered around the conditions for eligibility of providers to participate in the Medicare hospice benefit. Nearly everyone had some major objections to some portion of the regulations, but major objections were heard from small, volunteer-staffed hospices as well as hospitals. These hospices pointed out that they would never be able to offer the full range of services that were now mandated in order to participate in the Medicare hospice benefit, and as a result, they and the patients they served appeared to be excluded from the Medicare benefit. Hospitals believed that the conditions of eligibility favored home care hospice in that they allowed such programs to contract with hospitals for inpatient care but did not allow hospitals to contract for home nursing care. Hospitals had to provide such services themselves, in effect requiring hospitals to establish home health agencies. All of the hospice programs were concerned by a statement in the final regulations that said: "The hospice may not discharge, at its discretion, a patient whose care promises to be costly or inconvenient. Once a hospice chooses to admit a Medicare beneficiary, it may not discharge the patient." As a result of these concerns, fewer than 10 percent of the country's hospice programs had applied for certification under the final Medicare regulations as of January 1984.[56]

Table 5. Medicare Reimbursement Rates, 1983

Category of Service	Proposed Rates in August 1983, $ per day	Final Rates in December 1983, $ per day
Routine home care	53.17	45.48
Continuous home care	311.96	358.67
Inpatient general care	271.00	271.00
Inpatient respite care	61.65	55.33

Commentary

What can be said about the Medicare hospice benefit? What are the important points that can be made and that deserve to be watched in the future?

The inclusion of hospice services as a covered benefit under Medicare has irrevocably changed the hospice movement in the United States in a number of ways, some for the good and some to the possible detriment of that movement. For one thing, it has provided hospice programs with a steady stream of financing that will allow them to become stronger and more stable and to offer their patients a wider variety of high-quality services. For another, it has ensured that hospice programs are now an integral part of the American health care system, that they have been "accepted" in an important fiscal way. Finally, it has made vast numbers of Americans more actively aware of death and dying and of the special needs of terminally ill patients and their families.

Nevertheless, the passage of the Medicare hospice legislation has brought some disturbing negative effects as well. Whereas previously there was a prevailing spirit of enthusiastic voluntary participation by all persons involved with hospice and a belief that each individual's efforts were important to the program, there now is more concern with fiscal matters, administrative and management concerns, reimbursement issues, licensing, accreditation, and the like. The former spontaneous exuberance and personal involvement may still be there, but they are no longer the governing spirit in many hospice programs.

In addition, the matter of becoming eligible for Medicare participation has put greater emphasis on meeting standards, maintaining a qualified professional staff, and having the proper professional qualifications and procedures. Hospice has become more of a technical and professional service than it once was and runs the danger of becoming just another health service, rather than the unique personal service it has been. When a service is reimbursed under a health insurance plan, it perforce becomes a "health" service and perhaps less of a "human" service, in the broad sense.

Also, with the development of the Medicare hospice benefit and the acceptance of hospice care into the health care system, there is always the danger that hospice loses its independence, its ability to innovate, its creative iconoclasm that has made it so energetic in its development. "Joining the club" and submitting to a broad panoply of regulations and standards may permanently fix hospice care in a certain mold preferred by Medicare and may prematurely cut off further experimentation and development in the organization of hospice services.

Exactly what effect the results of the National Hospice Study will have on the implementation of the Medicare hospice benefit is unclear, but clearly it will be important. It seems apparent that hospice is not always a way to save money; further, it is apparent that there is wide variation in the use of hospice services and in the impact of those services on patients. Accordingly, it probably can be expected that Medicare will proceed slowly in expanding the benefit any further than at present. Indeed, it would seem more probable that Medicare will examine the National Hospice Study data to determine exactly which situations benefit patients and save Medicare money, and that Medicare will then try to direct the benefit more specifically and pointedly toward those situations in particular.

Summary and Commentary

Although hospice programs began only a few years ago as low-budget, relatively unsophisticated, volunteer-dependent organizations, they have begun to change considerably in the past few years. Hospices have begun to realize the necessity of a stable stream of long-term financing, have started to obtain considerable financial support from existing health insurance plans, and have been able to obtain congressional approval for hospice coverage under Medicare.

At the same time, until recently there have not been enough data to allow accurate and comparable measurement of the real costs of operating hospice programs and of providing the individual service elements that, taken together, comprise a hospice program. Until fairly recently, there have not been enough accurate data collected in a uniform manner to make meaningful comparisons possible among individual hospice programs of various models or between hospice programs in general and conventional forms of care.

The preliminary data from the National Hospice Study reflect wide variability among the various types of hospices in costs of providing care and indicate that hospice care does not always save money for the third-party payers such as Medicare. It is clear that certain types of hospice programs can benefit certain patients in some stages of their illness, but the ideal mixture of program, patient, and disease stage are not clear yet.

Even with the National Hospice Study, there is still no easy means of determining the total costs for an individual patient or for all dying patients without conducting a special study of the type recently completed by Lubitz, Gornick, and Prihoda for the Health Care Financing Administration.[57] Without easy access to the total costs of an illness (as opposed to the individual episodes of hospitalization, use of physicians, home care, nursing homes, and the like), it is difficult to measure the impact of hospice care on the total cost of illness and terminal care.

For public policy to advance in the area of hospice financing, a number of important steps may need to be taken, some rather quickly and others perhaps more slowly. Certainly, the results of the National Hospice Study need to be analyzed carefully and honestly and then put to work in planning the next stages of hospice development. This is clearly the best information that will be available regarding hospice care for many years to come, and the opportunity should not be lost to put it to vigorous use.

At the same time, the results of the early implementation of the hospice Medicare benefit need to be reviewed carefully as well. Even though the implementation of the hospice benefit may be uneven across the country and may be more reflective of home care hospices than hospital-based programs, it can provide a much broader data base than has been in existence up to this point and can be a valuable asset to future planning.

The process of accreditation, licensing, and standardization of hospice services that has already begun needs to be continued, so that greater uniformity and comparability exist among hospices and among the same hospice services provided by different types of programs. To parallel this, a uniform accounting system for hospice programs needs to be developed, so that more exact analyses of costs of hospice care can be carried out. Also, a more exact and accurate way of describing the severity of patients' illness is needed, so that comparisons can be made among patients with similar severity of illness and need for service. Without these standardized methods of describing hospice services, hospice finances, and hospice patients, comparisons among hospice programs or between hospice programs and conventional care will be pointless and, perhaps worse, misleading.

Finally, a better way is needed of aggregating the total costs of providing care over the entire course of illness for patients dying with cancer, so that the proper role of hospice care within the total sequence of care can be better understood. If the real impact of hospice care on the cost of terminal illness is ever to be known, these broader data will have to become known and made more readily accessible than they are now.

Hospice programs have moved quickly to establish themselves as important resources for desperately sick patients. If they are to continue to play an important role in the care of the terminally ill, considerable attention will have to be given to the exact manner in which financial support is provided to the programs and their patients.

References

1. Congressional Budget Office. Cost Estimate, Bill No. H.R. 5180. Bill title: A bill to amend Title XVIII of the Social Security Act to provide the coverage of hospice care under the Medicare program. June 25, 1982.

2. Department of National Health and Welfare. Policy, Planning, and Information Branch. *Palliative Care in Canada.* Ottawa, Canada: DNHW, 1982 Sept.

3. Congressional Budget Office.

4. General Accounting Office. *Report to the Congress: Hospice Care—A Growing Concept in the United States* (HRD-79-50). Washington, DC: U.S. Government Printing Office, 1979.

5. National Hospice Organization, Health Services Foundation, and Hospital Research and Educational Trust. Delivery and payment of hospice services: Investigative study. Final report, 1979 Sept.

6. California Department of Health Services. Palliative care service pilot project. Report to the 1980 California legislature on the hospice project, pursuant to Assembly Bill 1586, CH 1324, 1978, Sacramento, 1980.

7. Buckingham, R. W., and Lupu, D. A comparative study of hospice services in the United States. *American Journal of Public Health.* 1982 May. 72(5):455-63.

8. Falknor, P., and Kugler, D. JCAH hospice project, interim report: Phase I. Mimeo, Joint Commission on Accreditation of Hospitals, Chicago, 1981 July.

9. Greer, D., Mor, V., and others. Evaluating the impact of hospice care: The National Hospice Study design. Mimeo, presented at 109th annual meeting, American Public Health Association, Los Angeles, 1981 Nov. 4.

10. Lack, S., and Buckingham, R. *First American Hospice: Three Years of Home Care.* New Haven, CT: Hospice, Inc., 1978.

11. Johnson-Hurzeler, R. Speech by administrator of Connecticut Hospice at National Hospice Organization annual meeting, 1982.

12. Sweetser, C. Integrated care: The hospital-based hospice. *Quality Review Bulletin.* 1979. 5(5):18-22.

13. Outpatient hospice program decreases cost, maintains quality. *Hospital Peer Review.* 1981 July. pp. 78-81.

14. Van de Creek, L. A home care hospice profile: Description, evaluation, and cost analysis. *The Journal of Family Practice.* 1982. 14(1):53-58.

15. Carney, K., and Burns, N. Hospice care: A case study. Working paper, series no. 82-11, preliminary draft, Department of Economics, College of Business Administration, University of Texas at Arlington, 1982.

16. Carney, K. An economic perspective on hospices. In: Musacchio, R. A., and Hough, D. A., editors. *Socioeconomic Issues of Health, 1981.* Chicago: Center for Health Policy Research, American Medical Association, 1981, pp. 93-107.

17. Bloom, B., and Kissick, P. Home and hospital cost of terminal illness. *Medical Care*. 1980 May. 18(5):560-64.

18. Kassakian, M., Bailey, I., and others. The cost and quality of dying: A comparison of home and hospital. *Nurse Practitioner*. 1979 Jan.-Feb. 4(1):18-23.

19. *Palliative Care Service Pilot Project, January 1975 to January 1976*. Montreal, Canada: Royal Victoria Hospital, McGill University, 1976.

20. Walter, N. Hospice Pilot Project Report. Hayward, CA: Kaiser-Permanente Medical Center, 1979.

21. Cummings, M. A., Mundell, M. B., and others. A cost comparison study of hospice and nonhospice terminal care. Working paper, Kaiser-Permanente Medical Care Program, Los Angeles, 1982 Mar.

22. Kay, L. L., Cummings, M. A., and Mundell, M. B. Hospice: A cost analysis of three programs. Kaiser-Permanente Medical Care Program, Southern California Region. Funded by National Cancer Institute, Contract No. 85375, 1981 July.

23. Gravely, G., and Breindel, C. Costs of providing a mixed-unit hospice program. Unpublished paper, Department of Health Administration, Medical College of Virginia, Virginia Commonwealth University, 1980 July.

24. Amado, A., Cronk, B., and Mileo, R. Cost of terminal care: Home hospice vs. hospital. *Nursing Outlook*. 1979 Aug. pp. 522-26.

25. Hansen, M., and Evashwick, C. Hospice: Staffing and cost implications of home health agencies. *Home Health Care Services Quarterly*. 1981 Spring. 2(1):61-81.

26. Van Buren, L. Hospice home care: A cost analysis of a sample of patients seen during 1980. *Home Health Review*. 1981 Sept. 4(2):10-13.

27. Tucker, J. L. *Hospice Pilot Program Evaluation of 3-1/2 Years' Experience*. Washington, DC: Health Care Planning and Research Department, Group Hospitalization, Inc., 1982 May.

28. Wilson, B. P., Blosse, R. W., and others. Hospice care: Perspectives on a Blue Cross Plan's community pilot program. *Inquiry*. 20:322-27. 1983 Winter.

29. Brooks, C. H., and Smyth-Staruch, K. Hospice home care cost savings to third-party insurers. *Medical Care*. 22(8). 1984 Aug. In press.

30. Kane, R., Wales, J., and others. A randomized controlled trial of hospice care. *Lancet*. 1984 April 21. 1(8382):890-94.

31. Greer, D. and others. *A Preliminary Final Report of the National Hospice Study*. Providence, RI: Brown University, 1983.

32. Birnbaum, H., and Kidder, D. What does hospice cost? *American Journal of Public Health*. 1984 July. 74:689-97.

33. Greer, Mor, and others. Evaluating the impact of hospice care.

34. Greer, D., Mor, V., and others. National Hospice Study analysis plan. *Journal of Chronic Diseases*. 1983. 36:737-80.

35. Mor, V., and Birnbaum, H. Medicare legislation for hospice care: Implications of National Hospice Study data. *Health Affairs*. 1983 Summer. 2(2):80-90.

36. Mor, V., and Hiris, J. Determinants of the site of death among hospice cancer patients. *Journal of Health and Social Behavior.* 1983. 24:375-85.

37. Birnbaum, H., Kidder, and others. Hospice costs under the National Hospice Study. In: Greer, D. and others. *A Preliminary Final Report of the National Hospice Study.* Providence, RI: Brown University, 1983.

38. Birnbaum and Kidder. What does hospice cost?

39. Cohen, K. *Hospice: Prescription for Terminal Care.* Germantown, MD: Aspen Systems Corporation, 1979.

40. Berger-Friedman, P., and O'Hara, T. Hospice reimbursement study. Frank B. Hall Consulting Company, Briarcliff Manor, NY, 1982 Oct.

41. Blue Cross and Blue Shield Associations. Initial statement on hospice care and payment for hospice services. Mimeo, approved Nov. 8, 1978, by the board of Blue Cross and Blue Shield Associations, Chicago.

42. Mulstein, S., consultant, Health Policy Benefits Implementation, Health Care Services, Blue Cross and Blue Shield Associations. Written communications, 1982 Feb.

43. Amado, Cronk, and Mileo.

44. Tucker.

45. The Tax Equity and Fiscal Responsibility Act of 1982, Sec. 122. Public Law 97-248, Congress of the United States.

46. Lubitz, J., Gornick, M., and Prihoda, R. *Use and Costs of Medicare Services in the Last Year of Life.* Washington, DC: Department of Health and Human Services, Health Care Financing Administration, 1981.

47. *A Summary and Statement of Conclusions of Cost and Fiscal Impact Analysis of Proposed National Hospice Reimbursement Bill.* Washington, DC: Health Policy Alternatives, Inc., 1981 Nov.

48. H.R. 5180, 97th Congress of the United States (1st session). To amend Title XVIII of the Social Security Act to provide the coverage of hospice care under the Medicare program. Panetta, L., Pepper, C., Waxman, H., Rangel, C., Gephardt, R., Conable, B., Gradison, W., and Madigan, E., 1981 Dec. 11.

49. Willging, P. Testimony before Health Subcommittee of the House Ways and Means Committee of the U.S. Congress, 1982 Mar. 18.

50. Hollander, N., and Ehrenfreid, D. Reimbursing hospice care: A Blue Cross and Blue Shield perspective. *Hospital Progress.* 76:54-56. 1979 Mar.

51. Hollander, N. Testimony before Health Subcommittee of the House Ways and Means Committee of the U.S. Congress, 1982 Mar. 18.

52. Congressional Budget Office.

53. The Tax Equity and Fiscal Responsibility Act of 1982.

54. *Medicare and Medicaid Guide.* Chicago: Commerce Clearing House, 1983 Aug. 400:10,144-97.

55. Medicare program: Hospice care. *Federal Register.* 1983 Dec. 16. 48:56008-36.

56. National Association for Home Care. Report, National Association for Home Care, Washington, DC, 1983 Dec. 20.

57. Lubitz, Gornick, and Prihoda.

Chapter 9

Hospices and Health Planning: How Many Hospices Are Needed?

Paul R. Torrens, M.D., M.P.H.

A major characteristic of the hospice movement in the United States and around the world has been the suddenness of its development and the rapidity with which it has expanded. In the late 1960s, there were possibly a dozen major hospice programs around the world; fifteen years later, there are apparently at least 1,200 in the United States alone.[1]

This surge in development of hospice programs has released a tremendous amount of pent-up frustration with the traditional methods of caring for the dying, a frustration that has been building and threatening to explode in some fashion for many years. Fortunately, the hospice movement has provided a constructive outlet for these previously unsatisfied frustrations and has given to the health care system a new and impressive program of patient care.

Unfortunately, this sudden burst of energy, this sudden growth of new programs for the dying, has been so quick and explosive that there has not been adequate time to do the planning that should accompany the development of a new range of services of this magnitude and importance. It can easily be said that hospice programs have just happened without much benefit of advance thinking and planning as to how they should happen. This rapid and relatively unplanned growth has had good and bad effects, both of which need to be considered.

On the positive side, the suddenness of development of most of the programs and the lack of formalized planning has been a good thing in that it has allowed the hospice developers to be unrestrained in their thinking by any previous models or any previously identified restraints. Hospice developers have been able to generate tremendous enthusiasm, harness that enthusiasm to a particular project, and try it out without going through any of the more formal planning procedures that other health programs have had to encounter. If it had been necessary for them to go through these steps, the process could easily have dampened the enthusiasm, demanded formal planning skills that simply were not available in the groups proposing the hospice programs, and delayed or prevented the creation of these new programs. If more formal and organized planning processes had been an essential ingredient in the development of hospice programs in the United States, there would probably be far fewer such programs today, and the hospice movement would not have the strength and vitality it does.

However, there have also been some negative effects that should be considered as well. Certainly a number of programs were developed without adequate resources or without clearly identified purposes and objectives. Most probably, a number of programs were overly ambitious for the needs of their communities or did not have a clear understanding of what was needed or possible in their communities. Finally, in many instances, attempts have not been made to determine how the new hospice programs would cooperate with and be integrated into the already existing parts of the health care system.

Up to now, it appears that the positive aspects of the hospice movement's development have far outweighed the negative effects of the lack of planning. For the future, however, as the existing programs begin to seek government and health insurance reimbursement, as new hospice programs begin to develop in a much more competitive environment, and as our society begins to review these new programs in a more detached and objective manner, the appropriate planning becomes more important, indeed essential, for the general health system, the hospice programs and the hospice movement itself, and the patients they are all intended to serve.

Background

Before discussing the specifics of the planning of hospice programs, it is important to identify some crucial background elements and some very important practical aspects of hospice programs about which all planners should be aware.

First of all, it should be understood that the term *hospice* does not mean the same thing to all people using that term. Therefore, if a person or a group begins to talk about planning a hospice, it is important to ask immediately, "What do you mean when you use the term *hospice*? Are you talking about an inpatient program, a home-care program, a combination of the two, or something else entirely? What specific items of service will be included in your program (such as inpatient care, pain control, bereavement counseling, homemaker services, transportation, legal advice, and the like)? Will the proposed hospice program provide all of the services itself or will it contract with other programs or agencies to make specific services available?" It cannot be assumed that the term *hospice* as used in the United States has any more definitive function than to make explicit that the program is dealing with the care of the dying. Specific definitions and minimum standards for hospice programs have been promulgated by the National Hospice Organization and other national or international groups, but this does not ensure that all people are using the term correctly when they speak of hospice.

In the same fashion, anyone approaching the task of hospice planning must eventually face the lack of clear and acceptable definitions for many of the basic ideas and features of hospice programs. Although everyone agrees that hospice programs deal with dying patients and that they provide terminal care, the definition of a dying patient varies widely and that of terminal care even more so. The concept of pain control is basic to hospice care, but when is pain really controlled — when there is absolutely no pain ever, 90 percent of the time, or 75 percent of the time? Does the concept of pain control vary with the type and location of the cancer, or does the definition change as patients get closer to death? All of these concerns may seem trivial to busy hospice clinicians, but to hospice planners, they are central to their task, and the absence of adequate definitions makes their work more difficult.

A third general background issue that must be faced is that very little, if any, useful objective data can be obtained and simply inserted into some standard planning formula. As one observer has noted, "The first thing a planner will notice in studying the hospice literature is the lack of measurable characteristics, the lack of statistical data reported, and the lack of clear guidelines for describing services or projecting service needs."[2] With some exceptions, very little statistical data have been accumulated that adequately describe a range of hospice programs and their services, or their cost, utilization, and results. Hospice planners at the present time will find it difficult to obtain sufficiently rigorous data on which accurate projections can be based.

Finally, even if the data were being gathered and published, it is doubtful whether the experiences of any two hospice programs in the United States today are directly comparable, because there is no standard model and because no two hospice programs in the United States are totally alike. The range of services offered, the definitions of those services, the manner in which finances of the program are aggregated and described, the types of patients admitted, and the stage of severity of their illness — all these vary so markedly from hospice to hospice that only general comparisons between one program and another can be made. Perhaps as more standardized models develop and as more standardized systems of definitions and data collection emerge, this comparability of data will improve, but for the present, it would be very unwise for any hospice program to plan its future on the basis of some other hospice program's data, unless all of the aspects of that other hospice program are well known and understood by the program doing the planning.

Why Bother with Hospice Planning?

Given the difficulties and the uncertainties of hospice planning, the lack of exact and generally accepted definitions, and the wide variety of organization formats, one might ask, "Why bother with more formal planning of hospice programs? We've done quite well without planning up to this point; why start now?" Unfortunately, national events have overtaken the hospice field and there is no longer any choice in the matter. Hospice programs must be more carefully and intentionally planned for a number of very good reasons.

The first reason is related to the financing of hospices. Although many hospices in the United States began as volunteer-staffed, low-budget endeavors, few of them have remained that way for long. As they grow, they require greater financial resources and more careful financial planning if they are to survive. A hospice staffed by volunteers who work out of a church basement, using borrowed telephone services, doesn't really have to worry too much about its financial future; a more developed program with a professional staff of 15 workers providing 24-hour services and coverage to several hundred families a year most certainly does.

Also, a rapidly increasing portion of the financial support for hospice comes from third-party payers, particularly the federal government. These large insurance carriers want to know that the organizations receiving their funds are using them as wisely as possible and obtaining the maximum effects from the funds. They also need to know what the hospices will cost in the future and what their need for financial support will be so that they (the third parties) can prepare to have those amounts available when needed by means of appropriate premium structures.

Another significant reason for carrying out careful hospice planning is the potential overproliferation of hospice programs with the resultant reduced occupancy, weakened financial status, and divided community support for each of the competing units. For example, the 1983 programs roster of the Hospice Organization of Southern California lists five separate programs in Ventura, a city of 55,000 people.[3] Although each of these programs may have a very legitimate reason for its existence, an objective observer might ask whether dying patients in that small city might have been better served by some single joint effort among the various groups.

The most pressing reason for better hospice planning is to identify

more accurately a community's real need for terminal care and to determine more exactly the most effective way to meet that need. Without that
intentional effort to document what needs exist and without examining
all of the possible options and methods of responding to those needs, programs may be developed that are misplaced, incomplete, poorly focused,
or otherwise inadequate for dying patients in that community. Such programs may also have the effect of drawing off professional or lay staff
who could be more effective if employed elsewhere. More programs do
not necessarily mean better programs for hospice patients.

Finally, it should be noted that careful hospice planning is necessary
to ensure that the proposed program is well integrated into the existing
health care system. Hospice programs should have good relations and communications with the doctors and the hospitals in a community, in order
to ensure early and appropriate referrals to patients, easy access to the
various provider services that the hospices need, and continuous contact with new ideas and new techniques in patient care. All of these relationships, communications, and cooperative efforts are made immensely
easier by careful hospice planning and by the intentional involvement
of these other parts of the health care system early in the planning
process.

The relationship between planning and the development of hospice
programs can be addressed on three levels. The first is institutional planning for individual hospice programs and requires the kind of planning
that a particular program must carry out if it is to develop, prosper, and
reach the goals it has set for itself. The second is areawide planning, which
requires an exploration of the issues that a community must face in determining how many hospice programs it needs, what types or models should
be encouraged, and what kinds of interactions the program should have
with the rest of the health care system. The third level is a national review
dealing with the need for hospice care and for specific types of personnel
and a further exploration of the financial implications. Each of these levels
will be examined in more detail.

Institutional Planning for Hospice Programs

Any group proposing to start a hospice program or other form of care
for dying patients should move through an organized process of planning
that examines the reasons for proposing the program, that tries to determine the need for such a program, and that reviews what is already being
done in the community.

It must consider what type of hospice program will best suit its purposes, must review the resources that are available for the program,

and must create a phased plan of development for the proposed program.

Examination of Motives

The first step in planning for a potential hospice program is to ask, "Why are we proposing this program? What do we intend to accomplish with this program? How do we see this program operating once it gets started?" Experience has shown that each person, each organization, and each group of interests that participate in hospice planning often has a different view of what the program will be, how it will operate, and what the end results will be. Very often, these differences are hidden until the program begins to operate, at which time they emerge to create confusion or dissension.

For example, a physician oncologist may want to start a hospice program as a better means of controlling pain and may view such a program primarily as a support for his or her medical work. Nurses may see the program as a means of improving the nursing care of cancer patients over the long term and may expect nursing issues to be the most important. Social workers, psychologists, and clergy may be more interested in the social, psychological, or spiritual aspects of terminal care, whereas a hospital or organization administrator may see it as a way of keeping beds filled, enhancing revenues, offering a new product to the community, or expanding the reputation and status of the sponsoring institution or program. Community leaders may see the new program as a means of getting away from professional domination altogether and may have a model of a program in mind that is not a health care or medical program at all, either in concept or in control.

Some people may be more interested in an inpatient program, others in a home care program, whereas some may be interested in cancer patients and others in a wider variety of clinical conditions. It is entirely possible that the proposed program can, in fact, meet all the various different expectations, but an active, vigorous, open discussion of these expectations must take place in advance, if problems are not to emerge later.

Being Prepared to Discontinue

No hospice planning effort should begin unless all parties are prepared to discontinue the proposed program as being either unnecessary or too difficult to carry out successfully. Very often, the early proponents of a hospice program are so determined to have a program (sometimes *any* program) that they avoid acknowledging real problems and put aside difficulties that should be considered more carefully. This is not to suggest that hospice planners should be scared off by the difficulties of starting a new program, but to suggest that no one who is unwilling to admit that the program is not needed, not practical, or simply not viable at that time should start planning a hospice program. Accordingly, the planning process must respect and indeed encourage dissent, must intentionally include representatives of multiple viewpoints, and must have the stated policy that a negative outcome to the planning process (that is, a decision *not* to proceed with a program) is as legitimate an outcome of that process as a positive one (that is, a decision to proceed).

Determination of Need

The next step — and one of the most important steps in the entire hospice planning process — is the determination of the need for the hospice program in that institution or community. As a start, the planners will need to know the number of deaths occurring in the community to be served and the percentage of these deaths due to cancers of various kinds. If the planners of the proposed hospice intend to care for dying patients with diagnoses other than cancer, as has been suggested in the earlier chapters of this book, data on deaths from those diagnoses must be collected as well. For the present, it is probably satisfactory to use the cancer death rate as the basis for the majority of the planning effort, because previous experience has shown that more than 90 percent of the initial patients of a hospice program will be patients with cancer.

Once information on the number of cancer deaths and the types of cancer (that is, the site of the cancer or the organ involved) has been obtained, then information about the actual circumstances of these deaths should be obtained in order to determine how many of the cancer deaths might be categorized as difficult deaths and how many of the patients might have benefited from the types of services that hospices traditionally offer. It is important to know how many of the deaths occurred in hospital and how many at home, how many of the dying patients had home care and other forms of support, and how many were left virtually alone.

One way to obtain this information is by a questionnaire or a direct survey of persons who have been associated with dying cancer patients during the preceding year — physicians, nurses, social workers, priests and ministers, relatives of patients who have died, administrators of hospitals and home care programs, and others who can give accurate information from which an estimate can be made of the number of difficult deaths or deaths that should be served by a hospice program. Included in this questionnaire and survey process should be health care professionals who are at present caring for dying patients and families of dying patients.

From this process, the planners should have a fairly accurate estimate of the number of patients with cancer who can be expected to die each year in the community to be served by the proposed hospice, and enough information to make accurate appraisals of how difficult those cancer deaths have been for the patients and their families.

At this point, the planning group will have to decide what proportion of the cancer deaths in the community the proposed hospice will try to serve (or what proportion of all deaths in the community, if that is the course that has been decided on). This decision will have to be based on a clear statement of philosophy with regard to the hospice itself. As noted in chapter 4, very different philosophies may be expressed concerning the types of dying patients that a hospice should serve—from one stating that *all* cancer deaths are difficult and therefore *all* dying cancer patients should be served, to a much more conservative one stating that hospices should serve *only* those cancer patients who are dying a very difficult death and whose difficulties have not been relieved by already existing services. The first philosophy is one that calls for a large, extensive program with a broad community outreach, whereas the latter philosophy would call for a much more limited, much more intensive, and probably more inpatient-oriented hospice program.

There is no magic that allows a particular group of hospice planners to arrive at the appropriate percentage of cancer patients that they ought to be serving. Indeed, this judgment may in fact be determined by the types of available resources, rather than the real needs existing in the community. However, it is important that hospice planners first attempt to establish their philosophy of what types of patients and what types of deaths they wish to be concerned with, without reference to available resources. After they have decided what they would *like* to do, they can determine whether it is possible.

However this decision is handled (that is, which kinds of dying patients the hospice will serve), it is almost certainly the most critical decision that hospice planners will have to make. It is also a decision to which a major amount of effort must be devoted during the early phases of the planning process, because almost everything else that follows will hinge on the outcome of this decision.

Review of Available Community Resources

At the same time that the need for the proposed hospice program is being determined, an extensive effort should be made to review what is already available in the community and what resources could possibly be brought to bear in any new program of services to be developed. In particular, an accurate and well-documented description of the present process of dying with cancer in the community needs to be developed, so that the planners know in detail the situation as it actually exists.

For the first of these two efforts, the determination of present programs and resources, the planning group must systematically review the present status of hospitals, nursing homes, home care programs, homemaker services, medical care services, transportation services, social welfare agencies, and the like in their community. This review should lead to an extensive list of existing services that are currently being used or could be used for the care of dying patients. Information should include their cost accessibility and should describe any restrictions or standards for eligibility. If the hospice planning effort is taking place within an institution or a program already giving care, such as a hospital or a home health agency, a specific effort must be made to identify all the current resources in that institution or program and to document how completely these resources are being used.

As part of the survey of existing resources, interviews should be conducted with individuals connected with the various services, in order to get their opinions about the strengths and weaknesses of their programs. These persons should be openly and directly made aware of the purposes of the survey and should be asked whether they feel a hospice program for the care of the dying is needed. Their advice should be sought concerning the type of hospice program they feel would be of benefit to the community and the type of services that they think should be included, and they should be asked whether they would participate in such a program if one were established.

In particular, the physicians caring for dying cancer patients should be approached and surveyed concerning their opinions about the desirability of hospice services in the community and their willingness to participate in some type of hospice program if it should be developed. They should be carefully questioned concerning the services they feel are currently not available to their patients and which they might be willing to help obtain. They should particularly be asked if and when they would refer patients to a new hospice program such as the one being considered.

As a second part of this review of resources, some cooperative physicians and families of dying patients might be identified, in an attempt to follow the process of dying for a small sample of patients in the particular community under study. Although this procedure is particularly difficult and must be handled with great delicacy, it can be the most valuable aspect of the planning process for a hospice program.

Ideally, if the planning committee can obtain the cooperation of some of the physicians in the community and can obtain from them the names of families in which a member is dying, a member of the planning group with some professional status (such as a physician, social worker, nurse, or minister) might approach the family in question and explain what the planning group is trying to do. That person might then say, "We are trying to find out what can be done to help improve the care for patients like your (father, mother, sister, brother, husband, wife, and so forth) and your family. We would like to talk with you from time to time, to get your ideas about what might be of help to you and what might be missing." In this way, it might be possible for that member of the planning committee to follow a patient and a family through the dying process in the actual community to be served by the hospice and to observe at firsthand all aspects of the present network of care in that community.

It might be argued that this information could be better gathered from other sources and that patients and their families should not be subjected to the intrusive questions of some member of a planning committee. Unfortunately, experience has shown that a series of anecdotal reports from various care givers does not always give a complete picture of the process of dying from the point of view of the patient and family. Where this type of participant observation has been used as part of a planning process, it has resulted in a much more realistic and personal picture of the needs of patients and families in that community, and a much more appropriate hospice program has resulted.

At the end of this phase in the planning process, hospice planners should have a detailed description of the various programs of care existing in the community, as well as a list of the resources present within the sponsoring institution itself. They should also have a good understanding of the process of dying from cancer for patients in the community under study and a clear idea of the real problems that beset dying patients and their families in that community.

Matching Present Needs and Available Resources

The next step in the planning process is to match the currently available resources with the real needs that have been identified in the various survey efforts. A list of the kinds of services that should be available to dying patients in the community should be drawn up, as well as a list of the available services, together with a description of their strengths and weaknesses. An optimal list of services that should be available can be taken either from the National Hospice Organization guidelines for hospice programs, from the Joint Commission on Accreditation of Hospitals (JCAH) standards for hospice accreditation, or the Medicare conditions of participation. A list of services that are available could be compiled from the results of the community survey.

A comparison of these two lists will rapidly point out those services or programs that are not available or that are currently not functioning well. A review in detail of several case studies of individual patients and their families going through the dying process will also point out whatever difficulties or deficiencies may exist in the linkage or coordination of the currently available services for the dying.

For example, the survey of caregivers and the observation of patients and families may have identified a need for rapid telephone consultation and reassurance for families. It may have also identified a need for reassurance regarding admission to an inpatient unit for the last few days of life, as well as a need for occasional inpatient "respite" care, so that families can be relieved of their patient-care responsibilities for a few days. The need for psychological or psychiatric counseling in dealing with unfinished patient-family emotional matters may also have been pointed out.

At the same time, the review of available resources in the community may have shown that none of these needed services existed already and that each would have to be developed. Or, the review of available resources may have revealed that all of these services existed in the community but that there was no good way of coordinating them or of bringing them to an individual patient in a personal and integrated fashion.

From this comparison of the needed with the available services and from the review of the actual long-term care follow-up study, the real needs for specific hospice services in the community will become readily apparent and, in many cases, the best manner of meeting these needs will become equally clear. If the planning committee or group has done its job well, the documentation of the strengths and weaknesses of the present situation in the community should almost automatically begin to suggest the necessary programs that need to be added and even the necessary organizational vehicles for carrying them out.

It should be pointed, out, however, that it is exactly at this point that the preconceived ideas or preferences of the hospice program supporters will begin to exert themselves and may actually begin to subvert the planning process. Consciously or unconsciously, many people interested in hospice programs carry with them a model that they wish to see instituted, even before the actual needs of services in a community have been objectively determined. For example, they may firmly believe that a particular community really needs an inpatient hospice unit or a pain control program or a psychological counseling program on the basis of what they have seen in other communities or other countries. Very often, the predetermined models will not disappear in the face of well-documented evidence; they will merely be placed in the background, to be subtly reintroduced at a later time.

For these reasons, it is extremely important that hospice planners obtain as much factual information as possible about the real circumstances of dying in their community and then that they insist that the planning deliberations be guided by the facts and not by individuals' assumptions or preconceived ideas. There is no point in going through all of the information-gathering effort, if at the moment of decision about the types of services that are needed, the facts are put aside and other subjective opinions are used as the basis for decision.

At the end of this phase of the planning process, the planners should have a solid appraisal of the presently unmet needs in the community and a good idea of the various types of patient services that will be required to meet those needs.

Estimates of Volume of Services and Professional or Institutional Resources Needed

The next step is to develop more specific estimates of the volume of services that will be needed for patients in that community and the amount of professional staff time or inpatient resources that will be needed to deliver this volume of services.

For example, let us suppose that a large hospital has 300 patient deaths from cancer per year and that it desires to provide hospice care to all 300 of these patients. Utilizing the JCAH accreditation standards for hospices, the hospital determines that its hospice patients should have a complete array of services available, including inpatient care, home care, bereavement care, transportation, and respite care.

The hospice planning committee for this hospital begins to review all of the various services that will be required and attempts to estimate the specific volume of services needed for each of these parts of the hospice program. For example, the planning committee may want all 300 patients to have home nursing care available to them, and by inquiry to various experts, it may estimate that each patient will require 12 home visits during the course of his or her terminal illness, a total of 3,600 home visits per year. Again, after inquiry to experts, it may be determined that one home-care nurse can make 3 terminal-care visits per day, 15 per 5-day week, or 750 per 50-week year. Since a total of 3,600 home visits were estimated as being needed to provide the necessary home care for the dying patients, this would lead to a nursing staff requirement of almost five full-time home care nurses.

In the same fashion, the staff requirements for each of the individual services to be included in the hospice program can be estimated, and a tentative personnel requirement for the new hospice developed. Planners must be aware of the roughness of these estimates and must make explicit the assumptions they are using in each step of the process (for example, how many terminal-care visits a single home-care nurse can make per day or per week). The estimates themselves must be used with caution, but if applied properly, they can give a good general picture of what the future hospice will look like.

Financial Planning Estimates

Once the staffing requirements of the new hospice are known, attempts should be made to determine how much money it will take to support each hospice service. For example, if it was determined that almost five full-time nurses would be needed to adequately meet the home care needs of the hospital's 300 dying patients, and if the average salary and fringe benefits for a home-care nurse is $25,000 per year, it becomes obvious that at least $125,000 will be needed to provide that element of the new hospice's service, without any administrative or supervisory costs added. Similar estimates can be developed for each of the individual services to be provided by the hospice, and in this fashion, a rough estimate of the total annual budget can be developed.

At the same time, estimates must be developed regarding the level of financial support that will be available to meet this total financial requirement. Foundation grants, donations from families and institutions, fund-raising drives, health insurance benefits — all possible sources must be reviewed to reach some estimate of the income that will be available to support the proposed hospice. As with many other estimates, it is important to recognize how rough these income projections really are, so that the expected financial support is not mistakenly overstated.

Choice of Organizational Model

While the estimates of needed staff and financial resources are being developed, the hospice planners must also give serious consideration to the organizational form or model for the new program. Will the new hospice be a part of a larger organization, or will it be an entirely new organizational entity? Will the new hospice try to deliver all of the proposed services itself, or will it contract with some other agency for the delivery of certain services while it delivers others? Will the new hospice use an entirely salaried staff to do its work, an entirely volunteer staff, or some mix of the two?

These are not merely technical planning questions; rather, they are questions of major policy for the new hospices, because they will form the basis of many of the more routine planning estimates. Some of these policy questions cannot be decided until it is seen how much of a particular service is needed and how much it will cost, whereas other policy questions may be decided first and then a particular planning estimate follows. Regardless of which comes first, the planning estimate or the policy decisions about organizational form or model, these two activities are closely related and affect each other directly.

Feasibility Plan for Program Development

The final step in this planning effort is to bring all of these various data, estimates, and decisions together, and to create an orderly plan for the development of the new program. If certain services are to be initiated first and others added later, this fact needs to be specified. If a certain portion of the patient load is to be cared for in the first year and additional portions of the desired total added in subsequent years, this plan needs to be described. If certain portions of the proposed program are to be developed when certain amounts of money have been raised or guaranteed, with other services to be added later as new monies are raised, this plan needs to be laid out. In short, a blueprint and a timetable for the staged development of the new hospice needs to be written, so that all interested parties will know where the hospice is going, how it intends to get there, and when each step in the development will actually take place.

Areawide Health Planning and Hospice Programs

Just as individual institutions must plan their futures carefully with regard to hospice care, communities also need to engage in areawide planning for hospice programs. Earlier in this chapter it was noted that the 1983 list of hospice programs compiled by the Hospice Organization of Southern California showed five programs based in Ventura, California, a city of 55,000 people. The same list showed only three programs in San Diego, a city of more than one million people.[4] It seems obvious that better areawide planning for hospice programs is needed, not only to ensure that there will not be too many programs in one area but also to ensure that there will be enough programs in others. The role of areawide health planning in both the discouragement of unneeded programs and the positive encouragement of needed ones is as important for hospice services as it is for other types of health care.

Unfortunately, just when there is the greatest need for organized areawide planning for hospice programs, the previous federally supported health planning system in the United States is going into marked decline, making it unclear what type of health planning will exist in the future. It seems clear that our health care system will become increasingly complex and expensive, and areawide health planning will be urgently needed. Hospice advocates would be well advised to work as if areawide health planning of some sort will continue to exist, because it most probably will.

An early investigative study sponsored by the National Hospice Organization in 1977 indicated very little interaction between hospice programs and area planning agencies at that time,[5] and even though there was an attempt in 1979 to develop some guidelines to help planning agencies review hospice programs,[6] very little came of the effort. The Health Systems Agency of South Florida did attempt to develop criteria and standards for hospice programs in its area,[7] and the Illinois Health Facilities Planning Board, the state health planning agency, did the same for hospice programs in that state,[8] but their efforts were more the exception than the rule. In 1980, when Thoreen carried out a survey of existing health systems agencies for the St. Paul-Minneapolis Health Systems Agency, in order to see what HSAs were doing in hospice planning, he found that even in their prime, areawide health planning agencies had little effect on hospice programs.[9]

Thoreen sent a mail survey to 200 of the then-existing 202 health systems agencies in the United States, and 165 (82.5 percent) responded. Of the 165, 75 percent said that there were hospice programs giving care to the terminally ill in their region. However, 65 percent of the respondents said that the hospice programs had not applied for a certificate of need prior to developing their programs, even though 47 percent of the respondents said that providers were required to apply for such a certificate of need for a hospice program. Probably part of the reason for this lack of formal application for certificate of need was the fact that only 42 percent of the health systems agencies had written a section on hospice care for their overall health systems plan.

An almost universal interest in hospice care was shown by the 165 responding HSAs, and there seemed to be a strong feeling that eventually hospice care would have to be included in any areawide health plan that might develop. However, there was little evidence of any vigorous attempts at the time of the survey to consider hospice programs in the context of areawide planning for health services.

When areawide health planning becomes stronger again, what are the issues facing health planners who must consider hospice programs as a part of their overall plan? What are the questions they must ask and the processes they must go through in order to develop an areawide plan for hospice care?

In general, the area health planning agency will have to go through much of the same process that the individual institution goes through as it considers its own individual hospice. The major differences are that the health planning agency is generally considering the needs of a broader community than that included within one institutional program. Also, the health planning agency will not have the responsibility of actually establishing and attempting to finance an individual program.

The health planning agency's process should probably include the following steps: (1) determination of need in the area, (2) identification of present or potential future services and programs, (3) comparison of need with currently available or future hospice programs, (4) establishment of proposed optimal level of hospice services to handle the currently unmet need and to guide the development of future programs, (5) inclusion of the hospice projections and guidelines in the total health plan for all health care services in the area served, and (6) establishment of a means of working with present or potential groups interested in the development of hospice programs in the community.

As a preliminary to the development of its own planning process, the health planning agency or community group doing health planning for a wide area should reinforce the requirement that each prospective new hospice program engage in a formal institutional planning process as described in the preceding section of this chapter. Indeed, if each prospective new program does its own institutional planning well, much of the health planning agency's work will already be done and its own role will be made much easier. This does not mean that a health planning agency can abdicate its areawide responsibilities to the individual prospective program, but it does mean that the overall health planning process for the area will be made considerably stronger by an insistence on well-conducted institutional planning for each of the new programs.

Determination of Need

As with institutional planning, the first step in areawide planning is an attempt to determine the need for hospice services. This step will require the determining the average number of cancer deaths per year in the area under consideration, with a breakdown of the total number of deaths by sites and type of cancer, as well as some indication of the number of cancer patients dying at home or in the hospital. Death certificates for the area under study may be a good source for this information, but perhaps an easier source will be the records of the tumor boards of the various hospitals in the area. As was mentioned with institutional planning for hospice care, if the total number of cancer deaths can be ascertained, this figure will give a good indication of approximately 90 percent of the need or demand for hospice care; however, if patients dying from other conditions are to be included, obviously deaths from these additional causes will have to be determined as well.

Those developing an areawide plan for hospice services will have to determine what proportion of the total cancer deaths might appropriately need hospice services. Here again, interviews will have to be carried out with physicians, nurses, social workers, administrators of hospitals and home care programs, ministers, and others who regularly deal with and care for dying cancer patients and who can give some general estimates of the numbers of difficult deaths and the particular problems that are most troublesome to patients and families. As experience with hospice care increases around the country, published data that review the experience of individual hospice programs elsewhere will also be useful. The health planning agency will have to determine the percentage of cancer deaths that should have hospice services made available. Obviously, the composition of the panel of experts will be very important and should include representatives from as many perspectives as possible, to prevent the panel from being captured by one particular point of view.

It is particularly important in the planning agency's process, even more so than in the individual institution's planning process, that the focus be primarily on the need for individual services, without any consideration (at this point, at least) of the most useful organizational vehicle to deliver them. The planning agency should first identify the individual items of service that are needed by dying patients in its communities (for example, home care, bereavement services, transportation, and so forth) and only later consider what would be the best organizational vehicle for delivering these individual items of services.

Identification of Available Resources

The next step in the planning process is to determine the currently available level of care for each of the needed items of service identified. For each of these services, the planning agency must determine whether any currently existing organizations or groups are providing these kinds of services, or whether they could provide them if asked to do so. Here again, the expert panel that helped to describe the particular services needed by dying patients could also serve to evaluate whether the currently available programs of service are meeting those needs. Their work should include interviews with health care professionals in the community and also with families of patients that have died within the past year, to determine the satisfaction of these two groups with the present level of service available in the community.

Just as it was recommended that the institutional planners attempt to obtain a firsthand view of the integration of existing services, it is important for members of the expert panel or staff members of the planning agency itself to follow the care of patients dying with cancer, in order to get firsthand impressions of whether the individual services actually come together in some type of coordinated package or program. This experience will allow the planning agency to approach the problem of developing an areawide plan in a much more realistic fashion and to understand the problem of integration of individual services with greater clarity.

Appraisal of the Match between Current Needs and Current Resources, and Development of Long-Range Plans

Once the planning agency has identified the types and kinds of services that are needed by dying patients, and once it has determined the present availability of these services in the community, identifying the shortfall and the need for additional services becomes a fairly simple task. The problems, however, will come in (1) trying to identify what the appropriate levels of individual services might be for a particular community and (2) determining the best organizational vehicles or programs for delivering these services.

No fully adequate guidelines have been established to assist planning agencies in appraising the optimal level of individual services, such as home nursing care, bereavement services, inpatient care, and the like, because each existing program has defined *need* in a different way and has used different planning assumptions. Several studies in England[10,11] and in the United States[12] have attempted to project the need for inpatient beds, but each has produced rather different estimates. At least part of this difference was due to different circumstances in which the planning effort was carried out, but a large part of the difference was probably also due to the well-recognized lack of exactness in the present methods of forecasting need for health care in general, particularly home health services.[13,14]

Instead of a community's trying to adapt formulas from another community whose circumstances might be quite different, it is probably better for each community to develop its own guidelines, using the opinion of its own expert panel. Over time, the experiences of various hospice programs around the country will need to be accumulated, and some standard service/patient/population ratios will have to be developed. For the present, adequate data do not exist to establish these ratios, and each community health planning agency would be well advised to proceed slowly and carefully with its own particular needs.

Development of Specific Plan

The last step for a planning agency is the actual production of an areawide hospice plan (or at least a section on hospice care in the larger health systems plan for all health services in the area). The initial drafts of the areawide hospice plan should be widely circulated among hospice and nonhospice experts alike, in order to allow time for appropriate comment, criticism, and corrections of factual error. The various assumptions that were used in drawing up the estimates in the hospice plan should be made very clear, so that the basis for the final estimates will be well understood.

In contrast to other areawide plans that deal with well-established programs of health services, the areawide hospice plan will have to be modified and revised yearly as more information and experience are gained about hospice work, both in the immediate community under review and in the country in general. The initial versions of the hospice plan should clearly state that the target figures contained in the plan are estimates and will be modified as more experience is accumulated.

As part of this continuing, several-year process of developing a final area plan for hospice care, the planning agency should maintain a continuous liaison with the hospice experts and advocates in the area, to ensure that a dialogue between planners and hospice workers continues until a final plan is completed. In order to take advantage of the lessons learned by others, planners should carefully review hospice plans developed in other areas, such as the one put together by the hospice workers and health planners in Cleveland, Ohio,[15] or the three-hospital cooperative effort put together by the East Central Illinois Health Systems Agency.[16]

National Planning for Hospice Programs

Probably the most important arena in which careful hospice planning should take place is a national consideration of hospice programs. Unfortunately, it may also be at this level where careful, thoughtful hospice planning may be the most difficult to accomplish.

The national health system in the United States, as compared to many other national systems of care, does not have a structure that allows for careful consideration of health priorities in the country and a rational allocation of resources on the basis of those priorities. Instead, our system is characterized by a rather chaotic and sometimes tumultuous coming together of special interests in Washington, DC, each of which wants to influence national events to benefit its own particular interests. Health policy is made item by item, legislation by legislation, without any referral to a broader set of health priorities for the country as a whole.

Whatever control exists over the health care system of the country is generally carried out in the regulatory and financial systems of the country, neither of which was established for the purpose of setting rational priorities and creating a means of rational allocation of resources. Simply by default, for example, the Medicare program exerts as much control over the shape, size, and manner of functioning of the American health care system as any other agency of government, even though it was initially established only to pay bills and ensure financial protection to people over the age of 65. The lack of any more central or intentional national health planning structure has created a vacuum into which the Medicare program has been drawn, largely because of its power to promulgate conditions of participation in its program.

Because this situation is not likely to change in the near future, because the United States will most probably continue to have a fragmented central health planning structure (if, indeed, any at all), and because planning and control of the system will probably continue to rest with individual regulatory and financing agencies, it is not practical to talk about a planning process at the national level like the one discussed in the two previous sections. Instead, it is important to identify those national hospice issues that need to be considered by hospice planners, regulators, and financiers — wherever they happen to be located in the national structure.

Access to Hospice Care

The first key issue to consider is how easily and under what conditions people in the United States should have access to hospice care, and how much hospice care should be generally available to the population. This issue translates into the simpler question: Should all dying patients or only some have hospice care available? If only certain dying patients are to be included (such as those with intractable pain, or those with severe psychological difficulties, or those without any family member to care for them), these limitations need to be made explicit.

What Kinds of Hospice Care to Encourage

As was mentioned earlier, the term *hospice* in the United States now means a program of care for dying patients, a program that can be delivered through any one of a number of vehicles. Each type of organizational model has advantages as well as disadvantages, and so the question then becomes: Which model or type of hospice should be encouraged, if any? A model that stresses home care primarily and does not put much emphasis on inpatient care achieves a certain kind of result, whereas a model that focuses much of its energies on inpatient care and not so much on home care, achieves another. Each model has to be reviewed and a decision made as to which one, if any, is to be the preferred model.

Hospice as a Freestanding Program versus Hospice as an Integral Part of the Larger Health Care System

Hospice began, both in Great Britain and the United States, as a separate and somewhat independent movement, completely and wholly outside the established health care system. This independent status allowed it a freedom of movement and development that would not have been possible if it had been subject to the restraints of the larger health care system.

Now that the idea of hospice has been generally accepted, however, and now that hospice programs are being drawn more closely to the traditional health care system (and vice versa), the issue arises: How much independence from and how much integration with the traditional health care system should there be for hospice programs? Is the time appropriate now to bring all hospice programs totally and completely into the broader health care system and, in effect, do away with the refugee status of hospice care? Or, should hospices be encouraged to be as independent as possible, so that they continue to innovate and experiment, so that they continue to involve the vigorous energies of volunteer, non-health-professional leadership? There are advantages and disadvantages to the American people with each approach, and the issue must be addressed directly by national policymakers.

Hospice versus Other Demands for Health Care

Like other forms of health care, hospice is only one item in a much broader social agenda for health care in the United States. Not only do the American people need hospice care, they need improved services for mental illness, they need expanded services for stroke and other forms of disability, they need enhanced care for alcoholism and other forms of substance abuse—and on and on. Hospice advocates can no longer contend that the main social question is whether hospice care is worth offering to the people of this country. Now the social question is whether hospice care is as important as or more important than a number of other items that also need to be provided for the American people.

It is clear that this society is rapidly approaching the limits of what it can afford to spend on health care, including hospice care. Society must make difficult priority decisions about where and how our increasingly scarce financial resources should be spent. Hospice planners must be prepared to integrate hospice requirements for resources into the broader requirements for resources for health care in general, so that our most important health needs are met within a reasonably orderly set of priorities.

Need for Hospice Personnel

The lack of specifically trained personnel to work in the hospice programs has become more apparent with the development of more new programs. Nurses with special training in the care of the dying, experts in bereavement counseling, physicians with special interest and experience in pain control, managers who can cope with the unique organizational and financial arrangments of hospice programs — all these personnel are in very short supply.

This is not to say that the individual programs have not done yeoman work with the personnel that they have had available to them, but rather to say that they could (and would) do even better work if there was a larger body of trained and experienced personnel who could be brought into hospice programs throughout the country. This may mean that special training programs for the preparation of hospice workers may need to be established and funded through training and educational grants, special contracts, and other devices to assist in the development of a larger pool of trained personnel.

It will be necessary to carefully identify the special personnel needs of hospice programs now and for the future, determine how these personnel can best be trained and prepared for their work, and then develop plans to offer and finance that training. If hospice work is to flourish, it will need expert people to help in the work, and the planning for these personnel must be one of the most important priorities for hospice planners in the years ahead.

Insurance Coverage for Hospice Care

In a country in which most institutional care is covered by health insurance of one kind or another, it is important that the issue of insurance coverage for hospice care be carefully addressed. A first step has been taken by the addition of hospice benefits to most commercial insurance plans, and a further step has been taken by the extension of hospice coverage to Medicare recipients, even though this latter coverage remains somewhat confusing because of the complicated nature of the coverage itself.

For the future, planners both in government and private insurance organizations will have to consider hospice coverage from quite a different point of view, looking not so much at *whether* hospice benefits should be included but instead looking at *how* they might best be included, what type of benefits should be covered, and what particular population should be addressed. Financial and utilization data will have to be carefully collected and analyzed, various insurance options tried, and a variety of forms of coverage offered. Integration of hospice coverage with broader health insurance coverage must be carefully reviewed to ensure that the two coverages are continuous and complementary, not duplicative and competitive.

Capital Requirement for Hospice

Finally, those interested in hospice planning on the national level must consider the needs of capital financing for hospice care in the years to come. Although the structural needs of hospice programs have not been great thus far, it is clear that there will be needs for the construction of special inpatient units, the conversion of old units, and the development of new forms of accommodation for home care programs, day hospitals, group counseling centers, and the like. Planners must realize that hospice in the United States has been virtually free of capital requirements up to this point, but this circumstance will certainly not continue into the future. Careful and thoughtful planning must begin now, if hospices in the future are to have access to the capital finances that they will need to continue and expand their work as that work deserves.

Summary

Hospice programs have been fortunate up to this point to have flourished without the benefit of any organized planning. They have harnessed the massive energies of many people in many communities to the hospice effort and have moved ahead with an impressive momentum.

The lack of planning, however, has created problems in individual hospice programs, in communities, and in the country in general. Although these problems, which are only now beginning to become obvious, are not now of such a nature as to seriously threaten what has already been accomplished, the unplanned pattern of the past should not continue into the future.

The future of hospice work in the United States will require a much more careful and orderly approach to the development and support of hospice programs throughout the country than has been necessary in the past. Hospice workers will probably mourn the loss of the freedom of innovation that was present in the past, but they should also see that the development of strong, stable hospice programs in the future will depend on more careful planning—for individual programs, for their communities, and for the country as a whole.

References

1. Falknor, H. P., and Kugler, D. JCAH hospice project, interim report: Phase I. Mimeo, Joint Commission on Accreditation of Hospitals, Chicago, 1981 July.

2. Johns, L. Issues in planning for hospice services: An introduction. *Technical Assistance Memo 76.* San Francisco: Western Center for Health Planning, 1980 Dec. 31.

3. Hospice Organization of Southern California. Southern California hospice programs. Mimeo, HOSC, Los Angeles, 1982 Dec.

4. Hospice Organization of Southern California.

5. National Hospice Organization. Delivery and payment of hospice services: Investigative study. McLean, VA: NHO, 1977 Sept.

6. The development of guidelines for the HSA review and planning of hospice programs: Final report. Mimeo, prepared for the Health Systems Agency of Southeastern Pennsylvania by ELM Services, Inc., Washington, DC, 1979 May.

7. Health Systems Agency of South Florida. Criteria and standards for hospice (draft). Mimeo, Miami, FL, 1978.

8. Hatch, E., and Boring, N. Regional hospice network offers system benefits. *Hospital Progress.* 1980 Mar. 61:67-70.

9. Thoreen, P. W. Regional planning and review of hospice care: Results and discussion of a survey of U.S. Health Systems Agencies. Mimeo, Health Board of the Metropolitan Council, St. Paul-Minneapolis, 1980 Sept. 10.

10. Curnow, R., and MacFarlane, S. The provision of beds for terminal cancer patients in the catchment area of the Reading and district group of hospitals: Report to the working party. Operational Research Unit, Department of Applied Statistics, University of Reading, England, 1971 Apr.

11. Rugg, M., and Carr, A. The need for the provision of terminal care in Leicester and Leicestershire: Report to the Leicester Organization for the Relief of Suffering. Leicester, England, 1976 Oct.

12. Breindel, C., and Acree, C. Estimates of need for hospice services, *Death Education.* 1980 4:215-22.

13. Sharma, R. Forecasting need and demand for home health care: A selective review. *Public Health Reports.* 1980 95:572-79.

14. Harrington, M. Forecasting areawide demand for health care services: A critical review of major forecasting techniques and their application. *Inquiry.* 1977 14:254-68.

15. Metropolitan Health Planning Corporation. *A Plan for a Hospice System of Care for Cuyahoga, Geauga, Lake Lorain, and Medina Counties.* Cleveland, OH: MHPC, 1979.

16. Hatch and Boring.

Chapter 10

Ethical Issues Arising in Hospice Care

Joanne Lynn, M.D., M.A., and Marian Osterweis, Ph.D.

As the patterns of disease, the average life span, and the technologies available to intervene in disease processes have changed over the past few decades, the sensitivity and responsiveness of health care providers to the special needs and concerns of dying persons seem to have diminished.[1-5] Hospice care, as described in this book, takes an approach that is very different from the high-techology approach so characteristic of modern medicine. Instead, it focuses on providing for each patient as meaningful and comfortable a life as possible despite the fact that death is near at hand. Hospice providers have demonstrated remarkable and inspiring success in symptom control and in patient and family satisfaction.[6-10]

Although hospice programs have grown rapidly in number since their inception a decade ago, they serve only a tiny fraction of the two million people who die in this country each year.[11] The very success of hospice care in comforting dying persons has served to motivate advocates to try to increase the availability of these specialized services. However, it is just now becoming clear that there are a number of serious values dilemmas and choices entailed in the delivery of hospice services and in the organization of a hospice program of care and that these choices are made more pressing when the services are more prevalent.

As hospice evolves from a small, relatively private mode of care to a widely available, federally funded care option, ethical decisions that were once the province of the few persons directly affected will become the subject matter of policy decisions and practice routines. Private actions can be tolerated as long as they are not seriously harmful to defenseless persons or to the society generally. However, public policies must not only meet these criteria but must also maximally advance and protect widely held goals and values. Because resources are always finite, public policies must aim to be fair and equitable as well as protective of the rights and interests of individuals.

This chapter provides descriptions and some preliminary analysis of the major ethical issues that confront hospice caregivers and policymakers, including the range of treatment options that should be made available to dying patients, competent patients and the adequacy of consent, decisions to benefit incompetent patients, and equitable allocation of health care. This chapter will not treat the various legal problems possible or likely with a hospice care system, except as those issues arise incidental to the discussion of the ethical issues.

The chapter is predicated on an acceptance of three widely held moral principles: (a) patients should be primary decision makers, (b) informed consent is an essential element of ethically correct decisions, and (c) society is obliged to distribute health care in an equitable fashion. These and other strongly held values may often be of uncertain application and definition in a given setting and may sometimes be in sharp conflict with one another. Recognizing the potential for such values conflicts (or ethical dilemmas) and knowing how to resolve them is important both to optimal patient care and to responsible public policy. This chapter will illuminate these dilemmas, especially with regard to the effects of the currently pressing public policy decisions about hospice care.

Range of Treatment Options

What treatment options should be made available to dying patients? Are dying patients different from other patients in any important ways? Do any differences imply that some options should or should not be made available to them, both with regard to initial treatment options and with regard to decisions that arise during the course of therapy when some of the circumstances may include iatrogenic complications? In this section, the analysis will not extend to the effects of costs and resource use on the availability of treatment options. Rather, the inquiry is focused on what kinds of differences, if any, should exist in the treatment alternatives offered to a patient who is dying as distinguished from one who is not expected to die soon.

Why Is Life Not Considered a Terminal Illness?

Hospice programs are built on the conviction that a special kind of care is needed for those patients who are dying, implying in passing that this sort of care is not necessarily for those who are not dying. Sometimes this contention is phrased as the hospice commitment to "care" rather than the hospital's overwhelming concern for "cure."[12] When cure is no longer possible, the focus of care is said to change to symptom relief. This claim, which has been an important justification for hospice to be a separate and distinct kind of health care, requires being able to define the class "dying patients" in a clear way and to show that the patients thus defined are in relevant ways different from other patients. Neither requirement can be met.

For all patients, health care providers are obliged to use the available means to benefit the patient and, as far as possible, to do so on the patient's own terms.[13] Although usually this means to cure when that is a possibility, it need not. A person might be able to be cured of a deformity, for example, only at great cost in money, time, and suffering. For such a person, the obligation of health care providers might well be to ameliorate symptoms rather than to pursue a cure, exactly as hospice advocates claim is the case with dying patients. On the other hand, patients who will be dying soon may well sometimes need curative interventions. The person who has only a few months to live because of widespread bowel cancer does not thereby lose the opportunity to receive emergency treatment for a hemorrhage caused by an accident at work. These examples show that what matters is not whether the treatment is curative or symptomatic or whether the patient is expected to die soon; rather, the critical element is whether the treatment offered would actually be expected to benefit the patient. The expected length of life will ordinarily be one factor to consider, but it is often not the decisive one.

Part of the problem with efforts to treat dying patients differently from other persons is that it is notoriously difficult to define *terminal illness* or *dying patients*.[14] Living will statutes have astonishingly circular language, for example, "incurable injury, disease, or illness . . . where the application of life-sustaining procedures would serve only to artificially prolong the dying process."[15] Most people who sign such a document probably do not recognize that there are many incurable illnesses for which life-sustaining procedures only serve to prolong the dying process, yet life might be very meaningful or quite long. For example, the patient with diabetes is incurable and is exceedingly likely to die of the disease, yet insulin and other treatments are commonly considered indicated until very close to death.

Some statutes use the phrase "when death is imminent."[16] A survey of what California physicians understood by that term included times as long as five years.[17] The problem is not just one of misunderstanding or inattention. Rather, it is probably impossible to define *terminal* or *dying* in any workable way that is not simply arbitrary. Life, after all, fits easily into most of the sentences that we use to describe terminal disease, for example, (1) it is certain to end in death in the not very distant future, (2) all that medical treatment can do is to delay the inevitable death, and (3) it entails a good deal of suffering which is finally relieved only by death.

This makes it very difficult to establish a clear dividing line between being mortal and being terminally ill.

If, instead of looking for concrete defining characteristics such as objective extent of disease, one were to look for parameters of the patient's subjective experience regarding dying, one would have at least a relevant distinguishing characteristic — the degree to which dying is a priority concern for the patient. However, this is a thoroughly unworkable criterion upon which to base difference in care offered and given, as it is unavailable for evaluation by persons other than the patient and would require providing similar care to patients with vastly different objective health statuses.

Thus, one cannot justifiably hold that "dying patients" are regularly served best by having available certain treatment options that are not available to other patients. Symptom control should be part of the care of all patients, and pursuit of cure should not be ruled out just because the patient is not likely to live very long despite the attempt to cure.[18,19]

Commonly, hospices have been unwilling to accept a patient unless all "indicated" conventional curative treatments have been exhausted. To some extent, although hospice providers may well be unaware of this effect, this requirement protects hospices from being complicit in a patient's suicide. However, such a restriction also functions to limit a patient's authority to control treatment decisions so as to determine what will happen with his or her life and death. A particular patient might well be better served by having stopped seeking a cure before trying all options. Such a patient might be very averse to suffering, have little to live for, be concerned about the status of the surviving family's finances, or be devoutly trusting in God. How many options with what likelihood of success must a patient have tried and found to be unsuccessful before he or she is permitted to choose hospice care? One would not want to insist that in every case all potentially curative treatment must be exhausted, for that would negate the patient's authority to decide how to live his or her own life; yet, at the same time, one would not want to design a care setting that is so emotionally and financially attractive that patients are really unable to pursue aggressive and curative treatment options.

Iatrogenic Causes of Death

A second area that deserves thoughtful consideration concerns the kinds of treatment that should be utilized when a dying patient experiences iatrogenic complications which, untreated, result in increased likelihood of death. In a hospice, should such a patient be treated or allowed to die?

There are two general ways in which the actions of caregivers can be the cause of the patient's death. First, the risk to life can have been a well-recognized and considered part of the needed treatment such that

the patient's death, although not desired, is a recognized and accepted outcome of the best care choices. Sometimes, however, the patient's death
comes about from an unusual, unexpected, or erroneous effect of the care
given. For example, a patient might have an unexpected life-threatening
reaction to a drug, might have an accidental fall and break a hip, or might
have a first seizure during a bath. Even though the hospice patient might
well have come to terms with an expected death, unexpected complications of treatment may not have been among the things that the patient
was considering when the decision to focus on relieving symptoms was
discussed.

Also, death arising from an unexpected treatment complication affects
caregivers differently than deaths arising from the unalterable physical
condition of the patient. Understandably, when caregivers feel that their
treatment has caused suffering, they will usually want to return the patient
to the status prior to the complication if at all possible. Sometimes this
is simple and uncontroversial. However, sometimes this effort to respond
to the caregiver's desire to ameliorate the damages will conflict with the
wishes or best interests of the patient. A patient who is eager for surcease
from suffering may not want resuscitation attempts after an anaphylactic
reaction to a drug, preferring to die instead. Yet, a hospice provider would
be in a morally tenuous position if he or she were to make it easy to allow
patients to die from such errors, because accepting errors might make them
more common.

Hospitals can avoid some of these problems by having carefully considered and clearly stated policies concerning high risk procedures and by
discussing such policies with patients and their families when appropriate.[20] However, this remedy does not apply easily to the hospice setting
where the risks are largely those of ordinary nursing care. Although it
would probably be unwise to decide that no hospice patients should ever
have fractures set, it would be equally unwise to decide that all hospice
patients should have bones set when fractures arise from an iatrogenic
complication. Hospices could have some guidelines, however, as to how
such a decision should be made for any particular patient. Hospice
providers are probably in a better position than hospital providers to tem-
per a decision about whether to intervene with knowledge of the patient's
overall status and goals.

Symptom Control and Suicide, or When Is Morphine Murder?

A third question regarding the range of treatment options that should be
given to dying patients may prove to be especially troublesome: are
caregivers justified in providing palliative treatment if it is relatively certain that the treatment will prove to be a major cause of death? This question may arise, for example, when a patient's pain requires doses of

morphine that predispose to pneumonia or that decrease breathing. Under such circumstances, the physician or nurse may question whether providing the narcotic is morally and legally correct.

Patients who are respected, valued, treated with compassion, given effective symptom control, and helped to deal with spiritual and family matters are much less likely than other patients to want to die more quickly than necessary. However, being sick enough to die is often far from the most appealing mode of existence, and some patients may not find the endeavors available to them to be as meaningful as do others who actually find special understanding and peacefulness as they die. Some patients may even prefer to hasten their dying. Other patients who do not have strong preferences about the length of life may nevertheless have symptoms whose treatment shortens the patients' lives.[21-24]

Hospice providers claim that treatments aimed to control symptoms are different from suicide or murder,[25,26] but this is a somewhat surprisingly difficult claim to defend. If one were to shoot a patient or give him cyanide in order to relieve his pain, one would be held guilty of murder, and the fact of the patient having asked for this and of the murderer's motives being pure would not exculpate the act.[27-29] So, what is different about vigorous symptom control using conventional medical means? Usually, vigorous symptom control is not as likely to cause death as these more violent examples, but cases occur where death is virtually certain. Usually, the connection between the act and the death is more attenuated in medical actions than in acts conventionally construed as murder, but that construction of reality rests on a convention rather than a reliable and explicable difference in the nature of the act in question. Finally, the only real difference is that certain professionals have effectively but somewhat informally been granted the authority to risk life in certain socially defined ways in medical practice — ways that would be criminal if done by others.[30,31]

This is a thin reed. The distinction between murder (or suicide) and symptom control is ambiguous in a number of borderline cases. Two especially pointed examples of the sort of case that should occasion serious reflection are the patient dying with respiratory insufficiency and the patient dying with malnutrition or dehydration.

The patient with terminal insufficiency may well have no treatment available to relieve the sense of suffocation, except the administration of morphine (or drugs with similar effects) in doses sufficient to reduce respiratory efficiency. Doing this will often lead to a self-perpetuating coma from hypercarbia and then to death, somewhat earlier than the patient would have died untreated. Providing morphine in such a case is presented as the obviously correct course in British hospice literature,[32] and it does seem to be the most justifiable choice. However, the situation is so close to direct killing that it deserves a pause for careful consideration, for careful explication of why this should be tolerated although deliberate poisoning is not, and for critical examination of alternatives and motives by all caregivers, families, and patients.[33,34] If the provision of such doses of morphine were to be done in an unreflective way, without due concern for the seriousness of the decision, or by persons not trained and sanctioned for making the decision to risk life in this way, then the likelihood that the act will be seen as murder increases.[35-37]

The patient for whom a proximate cause of death is malnutrition or dehydration presents a very uncomfortable situation for caregivers. Providing food and water for those who cannot do so for themselves is a very strong obligation in most situations. To fail to do so and to allow a person to die seems not merely erroneous but outrageous. However, not all people who require medical means to provide food and water are benefited by the endeavor.[38] Patients who are close to death seem to die more comfortably if somewhat dehydrated and in negative nitrogen balance. For some patients, the procedures required in order to avert malnutrition and dehydration are so onerous that the benefits are meaningless. Hospice caregivers have been impressed that those patients who can continue to communicate through terminal illness rarely find any advantage to artificial feeding. Yet, when a patient cannot eat or drink, death is sure. Again, why is a choice not to artificially intervene acceptable and not murder? The answer must lie in the choice being demonstrably in the patient's interests, after due consideration by competent professionals.[39,40] Vigorous public discussion of these cases near the borderline would help to clarify and define the acceptable standard of practice and help ensure that bad practices, when they exist, would be prosecuted correctly and that defensible practices would be protected.

Competent Patients and Informed Consent

In order for patients to make fully binding decisions regarding health care, they must be acting voluntarily and without undue external influence, they must be adequately informed about their situations and the likely effects of various choices, and they must be competent to deliberate and choose in a way that is both reasonable and responsive to each patient's own values and concerns.[41] Each of these preconditions raises concerns in the context of hospice care, both because of the medical and emotional condition of the patient served and, increasingly, because of the constraints that are likely to be imposed by public policies.

Voluntary Choice

The influences that others have on the choices of a patient who is very ill are rarely overt—there are not often threats of violence or incarceration. However, the patient is very likely to be in an emotionally

vulnerable position and to feel largely out of control regarding significant elements of his or her life. In these circumstances, the patient is all
too easily manipulated into making choices that are not in character and
even to making choices that do not serve that patient's best interests.

For a patient to be able to make a voluntary choice, the patient must
be able to feel that the choice is truly his or her own and that he or she
is capable of having an effect on the world and on the course of treatment. The patient must not be subject to coercive choices, in which one
choice is made so unnecessarily desirable or undesirable by others who,
without concern for the patient's own values and goals, aim to exert a
strong effect on the decision. In order to avoid putative choices about
treatment being in fact coercive, the alternatives must not be unreasonably harsh, which includes that decision options should not generally entail
actual or perceived risks of abandonment.

Hospices have been very concerned with patients having control over
their lives and have tried to be sure that patients know they are coming
to a different kind of care setting, that they are likely to die soon, and
that no further treatment aimed at curing the illness is thought to be indicated. How effective this informing is in enabling the patient to act freely
in making a choice is uncertain but often limited in the following ways.
First, the patient is very ill and may well be unduly induced just by seeing
a compassionate caregiver and being treated respectfully, when much of
the person's experience with traditional care settings may have been perceived to have been degrading. Second, the care offered in hospice may
be much more appealing than hospital care because it is easier on the
family's emotions and finances. Now that hospice care of a rather extensive sort is to be covered under Medicare,[42] there will be an additional
inducement to accept a hospice program of care, and it will be an inducement that might cause patients to accept hospice care despite preferring
aggressive, long-shot tries at cure or longer life.

An additional constraint on the patient's voluntary choice arises in
the Medicare reimbursement requirement that a patient who elects to
receive hospice coverage and then decides to try additional treatment of
the "terminal condition," thereby loses the remainder of his or her currently effective hospice entitlement period, which may be as much as 90
days. Since hospice benefits are comprehensive, the value of the loss will
vary, depending on the patient's likely service needs; but even at the minimum payment, the patient will lose home care benefits of over $50 a day.[43]
For a patient with few resources, the prospect of losing home care benefits
worth $4,500 or more, especially if the patient has previously used most
of his or her regular lifetime reserve of Medicare benefits, will create quite
a substantial threshold barring serious reconsideration of reentry into the
usual health care system. While it is not in itself unethical to require persons to make hard choices about their care, it is obligatory on those who
design the system not to make such choices harder than is essential for

enabling the care system to meet its other obligations, such as improving health and apportioning benefits and burdens equitably.

Information Required for Valid Choice

For a patient to make a choice that should be honored by others, the patient needs to know what the choice entails. Various standards have been proposed regarding the extent of information disclosure required, but a reasonably comprehensive and persuasive formulation is the following:

> [H]ealth professionals should ensure that patients understand (1) their current medical status, including its likely course if no treatment is pursued; (2) the interventions that might be helpful to the patient, including a description of the procedures involved and the likelihood and effect of associated risks and benefits; and (3) in most cases, a professional opinion as to the best alternative. Each of these elements must be discussed in light of associated uncertainties. The purpose of such discussions is not to inundate patients with medical facts but rather to give them the information they need in order to assess options realistically and to choose the treatments most consonant with their own values and goals.[44]

The obligation to so inform patients and to ascertain that they really understand what their choices entail is not unique to hospice. However, given both the novelty of hospice and its divergence from what people have come to expect based on their experiences in hospitals, the tasks are perhaps more difficult. Adequately informing and ensuring understanding prior to admission are likely to be further complicated by the physical and emotional state of the patient.

Patients and their families will need to know not only what will be offered in a hospice program of care, but also what will not be available, and what they must surrender in terms of Medicare benefits for hospital care. However, the obligation is not in any way met by the simple ritual of signing a written form. The Medicare regulations[45] propose requiring that such a form be signed and will take its signing as evidence of satisfactory performance. This is too low and misleading a standard for hospices to accept. Adequately informing a patient, especially one who has other attractive options for care and treatment, is likely to be a much more ongoing endeavor and may always fall somewhat short of the ideal. A consent form may serve as a useful summary of discussion but should in no way be considered a substitute for discussion.[46]

How well informed the patient must be to make binding decisions once he or she is receiving hospice care would seem to be an easier question—after all, the patient has already decided what seems to be the most important question. However, this is much too superficial an analysis. The patient who decided that hospice care was the best option at a time when pain or exhaustion was overwhelming may need to be able to reconsider once these problems are treated. The patient who once was quite willing to have no more radiation treatment may feel different when a new bone metastasis leads to severe pain. Some patients may also want to have a voice in the treatment choices regarding such mundane things as the vigor with which constipation is treated and whether to treat an infection with antibiotics. Providing the information necessary to allow the patient to determine what will be done with the rest of his or her life will be a constant obligation of hospice caregivers. For some, this will be a natural and valued part of their jobs. For others, the notion that patients who are sick enough to die should be troubled with these very difficult and upsetting questions will be alien and the giving of information will be perfunctory or evaded.

Sometimes, caregivers describe some kinds of care as "extraordinary," as opposed to care that is "ordinary," or "passive," as opposed to care that is "active." However, these characterizations may actually be unhelpful or misleading in many difficult situations.[47-49] There are some active steps that are clearly warranted — giving morphine for severe pain even though risking an earlier death, for example. And some passive behaviors would be seriously wrong — negligent failure to treat a traumatically severed artery would be such a case. The "ordinary-extraordinary" distinction can be used as one way of stating the correct but troublesome considerations of burdensomeness and proportionate benefit,[50] but is more commonly used to indicate some sentiment about an "artificial" or "unusual" treatment not being obligatory. These latter definitions are certainly of no relevance to the determination of the patient's interests.

Given the concerns voiced above about the barriers to a patient choosing to reenter the traditional care system after an election into hospice care, situations will clearly arise where informing the patient about the options open to him or her will necessitate providing information about the effects on reimbursement eligibility. The provisions in the Medicare legislation and regulations are complex, and this obligation may well prove to be an especially uncomfortable and all too readily evaded responsibility.

Decision-Making Capacity

A competent patient is one who has sufficient capacity to make a decision that is in his or her own interests after having been adequately informed about what such a decision entails. The decision as to whether a patient should be considered to be competent requires assessing the patient's ability to understand the relevant information, to communicate with caregivers about it, and to reason about the available alternatives against a background of reasonably stable personal values and life goals.[51]

Competence, or decision-making capacity, can be determined only in the context of a particular decision, because one could be competent to make one treatment decision but not to make another. Generally, the greater the consequences of a particular decision, the more careful should be the assessment of competence. Thus, competence may be viewed not as an absolute quality that is either present or absent, but as a relative quality that is assessed in a context of particular decisions and capacities. A competence determination about a particular decision need not involve psychiatrists; indeed, it need not involve physicians except to the extent that the observations and assessments of these experts are germane to the layman's determination of whether the patient is sufficiently capable that he or she should bear the responsibility for the decision that is made.

Hospice programs should be in no unusual position relative to this sort of issue, but in fact they often are because of certain aspects of hospice practice. For example, as a result of great sympathy for the patient's condition, there is often a tendency to assume that a dying patient is incompetent, or at least less competent than a nondying patient. Conversely, there sometimes is the tendency to unreasonably lower the threshold of competency for the patient and to accept *any* expression of opinion by the patient as a sign of competency, even though this may not be the case. In some natural death acts, for example, the patient's being able to voice an objection to withdrawal of life-support is taken as evidence of competence and evidence that the previously signed advance directive should be rescinded.

Ideally, dying patients should be recognized as having the usual range of decision-making capacities and flaws. They should be protected from seriously erroneous decisions arising from feelings of powerlessness, misunderstandings of their situations, inabilities to reason, and unstable or undeveloped values and goals. However, they also need to be protected from the frustrations and other harms that arise from unwarranted paternalist interventions by others. Hospices, then, just like every other program of health care, will have to attend to the need to constantly consider the capacities of their patients as decision makers.

Hospices are in a particularly good position to work to enhance patient competence. By the time they come to hospice, many patients have lost the sense that they are personally effective and valued. Hospices can rekindle self-respect, which is central to the ability of the patient to be a collaborator in decision making. Many hospice patients come to the program with overuse of psychoactive medication or with mental confusion as a side effect of drugs used for somatic problems. Attentiveness to these issues may return many patients to competence.[52] Also, when the decision facing a patient is one as subjective and difficult as how and whether to live, the opportunity to consider the issues over time and with supportive and nonjudgmental friends, and to be able to do so at home or in another nonthreatening environment, may be of great value. Hospices, more than other forms of care for seriously ill patients, can provide that opportunity.

Much about the determination of capacity to decide is contestable because it is so difficult to give concrete, working definitions of the parameters of "adequacy" regarding decision-making capacity. On the one hand, individuals want to be free to make the major decisions about how to live their lives without the interference of powerful authorities, including the government. On the other hand, individuals would want to be protected from the untoward effects of decisions made while their abilities to reason, consider, and decide were seriously flawed.

No system of competence determination can decide all cases correctly, nor can one unambiguously determine what would have been a correct determination in each and every case. Thus, what health care providers must do is design a system that is defensible in that the errors it makes are as few and as mitigated as possible.

Incompetent Patients and Treatment Decisions

Incompetent patients suffer while dying in the same ways and with the same possibilities for amelioration of symptoms as competent patients. The same values that guide decision making for competent patients — promotion of well-being and respect for self-determination — should also guide decisions made by someone else on behalf of incompetent patients. The difficult issue is how to ensure that these values are respected. On the one hand, one must be cautious not to allow the preferences of others to be freely substituted for what is in the patient's best interests or for what the patient would have wanted if capable of deciding; on the other hand, one would not want to foreclose treatment options for those people who lack the capacity to make decisions. Here again, this dilemma is by no means unique to hospice care, but it is one that has only recently been recognized as troublesome.

Although hospices have sought to define the family as the unit of care, they have not been explicit as to how to resolve the dilemma that then arises when the best care for a patient conflicts with the wishes or the best interests of a family. All too often, it is easy to follow the wishes of a family when the patient is unable to voice his or her own preferences. This course leaves the patient without an advocate for his or her interests, however, and is thus not a defensible practice. Rather, the family should be encouraged to make decisions, insofar as possible, as the patient would have made them or, at least, to make them in the patient's interests. When families do not do so, there must be a procedure to follow that ensures protection of the patient's interests and a willingness to follow that procedure on the part of the caregivers.[53]

Some hospice programs have not been eager to care for patients who are incompetent. Sometimes the care burdens seem to be too great; sometimes the inability of the patient to engage in reflection is disheartening. This tendency may become much more prevalent under the Medicare hospice legislation,[54] because the regulations require that the initial election to hospice must be made by the patients themselves; during the second and third benefit periods, if a patient has become incompetent, a legal representative will be allowed to sign the election on the patient's behalf.[55]

If surrogate decision makers for incompetent patients are not permitted to make this decision, incompetent patients might thereby be barred from receiving hospice benefits under Medicare. It is clear that provision must eventually be made for the perfectly reasonable procedure of proxy decision making or for the patient to have made advance directives;[56] without this provision, there would be an unjustifiable denial of hospice benefits to appropriate patients simply on the basis of incompetence.

Hospices have not generally set forth explicit decision-making procedures. Although the safeguard of formal procedures may not have been needed when hospices were very small and almost entirely home care, the larger organizations and more impersonal procedures that are likely to arise under Medicare reimbursement may call for regular methods to ascertain that patient's rights and interests are being protected from unwarranted incursion by measures adopted for the efficient and profitable operation of the hospice program.

One procedure that seems to have much to recommend it is to establish institutional "ethics committees."[57] Such committees could be established for hospices providing services in any model, from home care to freestanding hospital. They would serve to ensure that persons with multiple perspectives and special skills would be regularly available to advise patients, families, and staff about difficult decisions. Experience with this approach is quite limited, even in hospitals, but it has the appeal of being flexible, inexpensive, educational, and protective of the patients. The only available alternative is for a large number of decisions involving incompetent patients to go to court. That prospect is so alien to hospice philosophy that its contemplation is difficult. Court processes are often slow, adversarial, costly, and public—all characteristics that would be painful for families and patients near death. Only the establishment of justifiable standards and defensible procedures regarding decision making for incompetent patients will prevent the slow drift toward court that has been apparent over the past few years in the rest of health care.[58,59]

Equity and Justice in the Allocation of Services

Ideally, society should be prepared so that differences in the receipt of benefits and in the bearing of burdens are fair. When some are entitled to a service that others are denied, one would want there to be clear, persuasive, and relevant reasons for these discrepancies. Traditionally, hospice programs in this country have had entry criteria that effectively limited most of their services to a population that is composed largely of middle-class, adult patients who are dying of cancer and who are surrounded by friends and family. Whom should hospice programs serve, especially now that hospice services, at least in part, are a Medicare benefit?

This question has two aspects. First, which patients should receive the benefits of hospice care? Second, what impact should hospice care have on the overall system of health care?

Equity in Access to Hospices

There is no one criterion that serves to define equity in regard to health care generally. Some considerations that are ordinarily legitimate include the need for care, the likelihood of benefit, and the proportionality between the benefits to be offered and the burdens to be borne, by the patient and others, in providing the care. Some benefits in a society are distributed by absolute equality, by past merit, by desert, or by ability to pay. None of these is generally useful in justifying the distribution of the important components of an adequate minimum of health care. An equal distribution would be insensitive to the large disparities in need; merit and desert are much more suited as primary principles in rewarding achievements that are under a person's control, principles that do not apply well to most ill health; and ability to pay is an especially cruel way to distribute those goods and services that are essential to a minimally decent life and range of opportunities.[60]

Thus, the first question will be whether hospice care is a component of an adequate minimum of health care that society should guarantee[61] or whether it is actually an amenity or frill whose allocation need not be so closely considered. The answer is not obvious. Certainly in the present context of health care, hospice commonly offers very important advantages for a dying patient. Yet, these advantages are not clearly of the magnitude that compels the society to see that they are generally available. They are not, for example, so centrally important as childhood immunizations and emergency transportation services. Hospices, rather, are the sort of borderline case whose social importance is quite correctly decided as a political matter. Hospice could have been left as an interesting and important aberration in the health care system — one that could teach others while serving a lucky few and one that need not be distributed in any particularly fair manner. However, this society, through the Congress, has decided that the sort of care that hospice provides is too valuable for this. Instead, it is to be made available to all Medicare beneficiaries as part of their societally defined "adequate level of health care."[62] Other third-party payers will probably follow suit, which will serve as our society's way of saying that hospice care is part of an adequate level of health care, which pooled public and private resources seek to guarantee for those who need it.

The ensuing questions, then, will be to define the appropriate population to receive the benefits, the scope of the benefit to be offered, and the distribution of the burden of paying for and providing the benefits.

Traditionally, hospices in this country have had multiple admission criteria that serve to limit the population who will receive benefits, often in order to guarantee that the organization can serve the most patients with their specialized skills. Many of these criteria have been included in the statute authorizing[63] and the drafted regulations giving shape to the Medicare coverage of hospice.[64] Other less explicit incentives on hospice programs, especially under Medicare, are also likely to affect the population receiving benefits. The major explicit admission criteria are these:

- Limited prognosis (6 months under Medicare and 3 to 12 months under other programs)
- Availability of a home and a 24-hour-per-day caregiver (not an explicit criterion for Medicare, but likely to be the outcome of emphasizing home care)
- No other curative therapy indicated

In addition, hospices have been generally committed to caring for patients until they die even if their financial resources are insufficient to pay for their care. The legislation requires this of hospices receiving Medicare funds. Although this does guarantee that hospice patients will not be abandoned in very poor condition when money runs out, it also provides an incentive for hospice programs not to admit patients who have any significant likelihood of using up their resources before they die.

Whom do current hospices serve? The overwhelming majority of hospice patients are now (and are likely to be under Medicare) dying of cancer. Virtually all hospice patients have homes with reasonably intact families, because the hospice emphasis on home care and a primary caregiver at the home makes it very unlikely that dying patients whose home or family resources are inadequate will be able to meet hospice requirements for home care. The caregiver requirement also makes it likely that the family has at least moderate wealth, in that it must be able to afford, for a rather indefinite period of time, for a family member to be home and not at work. The selection bias toward having an adequate income is further reinforced under Medicare (or any other program that prevents discharging a patient) by the incentive not to accept any patient who is likely to become a bad debt. So, hospices are likely to serve predominantly patients dying of cancer who have families with sufficient physical, emotional, and financial reserves to allow the patient to die at home.

In addition, Medicare will reimburse hospice programs at a fixed daily rate for each of four categories of care for each patient.[65] Under this plan, hospices will benefit if they can select patients in each care category that require the least services. A hospice that cares for 100 patients who require little care can provide good care and still make a profit. A hospice that instead is willing to take half of its load in patients who need extensive services, although still in the basic care range, may have more difficulty providing all the care needed and still balancing the books. Thus, Medicare patients that are financially attractive to hospices are likely to be those in need of relatively little care.

Should hospice services be limited to this population? In order to answer this question, one must be clear about what hospice care entails. Hospice services are characteristically delivered by an interdisciplinary team that seeks to provide comprehensive care to patients. The focus is on effective symptom control and on allowing the patient to define care goals while accepting that death is close at hand. Hospices typically are very labor-intensive and are more prone to use highly trained and committed personnel in the hands-on care than are typical traditional care models. These are valuable and relatively expensive services. Who needs them most and who can benefit most from such care?

There are many patients who are far from dying who would benefit greatly from most of the services that hospice programs offer. Many patients who are seriously debilitated or chronically ill would surely benefit as much as dying cancer patients from extremely attentive care and effective control of symptoms. Many of them also have spiritual, emotional, and family problems that could be helped with an energetic interdisciplinary approach. Hospice's emphasis on helping with the emotional turmoil of dying is a unique characteristic only if other programs of care are persistently unwilling to address these needs, and there is already substantial evidence of hospitals and physicians becoming more attuned to meeting these needs in a variety of care delivery settings.

Even if benefits providing for comprehensive symptom control are to be limited to the dying who are served by hospice programs, there is even less reason to limit the coverage to cancer patients with substantial resources in home and family. This serves to perpetuate a social inequity rather than redress it. The poor patient who has too few resources to die comfortably at home, or who has no home, is likely to be in greater need than the patient who will actually receive care under the current scheme. Similarly, the elderly patient, for whom the Medicare benefit is designed, is less likely than a younger patient to have a primary caregiver in the home. Even for the elderly patient with a spouse, the spouse may be too elderly and frail to provide care.

These poor and elderly patients are now cared for primarily in hospitals and in nursing homes. In hospitals, it is possible that they will be shunted aside as being of a lower priority for care than a potentially curable patient.[66-68] Also, because patients who are principally receiving symptom control are only a small part of the overall patient population, designing staffing and practice patterns to be responsive to these needs can be difficult and not financially rewarding. In nursing homes, the staff is likely to be too small in number and inadequately trained to provide effectively for the patient's subjective concerns and symptom control needs. Thus, the available alternatives to hospice care may be distinctly less desirable for a patient who is not wealthy enough, financially and emotionally, to qualify for hospice care.

Because health care is costly and because the need for care is highly unpredictable, largely beyond patient's control, and unevenly distributed among people, most individuals cannot make provisions for their health care without some mechanism for sharing costs with others.[69] This sharing of costs is done through private insurance and through government programs. Policies that restrict access to health care, including hospice, should be equitable and fair—they should not discriminate in arbitrary ways or distribute the costs of care unfairly. From the preceding discussion in this section, it is clear that hospice care under Medicare will be accessible only to limited categories of patients. Yet, because this is a federally funded program, all people are effectively paying for this service. Thus, not only do the admission criteria seem rather arbitrary, but the financial burdens are inequitably distributed relative to the benefit.

Impact of Hospices on the Health Care System

Hospices, especially with the advent of the new legislation, have the potential not only to be counter-redistributive but also counter-reformative. Some hospice advocates believe that hospice programs should aim to change the main health care system to become more responsive to the needs of dying patients. Their hope is that the hospice approach to care of terminally ill patients will result in a ripple effect into the rest of the system, thereby obviating the need for more special hospice programs.

Others claim that hospices are unique and uniquely beneficial to dying patients so that they should be available to all dying patients, and the regular health care system should be kept very separate from this specialized care of the dying. This latter claim not only seems unpersuasive theory, but it seems unwise on pragmatic grounds as well.[70, 71] Most patients will continue to die in traditional care settings, and those caregivers could become much more adept at caring for dying patients. The components of care in hospice are hardly so arcane that they could not be provided in traditional settings if doing so were a priority.

The selection biases and the structure of the Medicare benefit for hospice, however, reduce the likelihood that hospice will become a force for reform. First, the selection biases remove from the traditional care setting some of the most politically powerful patients—cancer patients with reasonable resources. Second, the Medicare legislation requires that hospices be substantially separate from traditional institutions, thus helping to create a specialization of function that makes it less likely that hospice services (or the hospice approach to the care of the dying) will grow in hospitals or that hospices will be able to use hospital facilities and expertise.

Finally, if hospices end up costing a substantial amount, as seems increasingly likely, then those resources are likely to come from other programs whose beneficiaries are less powerful or whose benefits are more discretionary. Because hospice benefits under Medicare come from the same funds as those that supply medical benefits to the elderly generally, this creates the distinct possibility that hospice will serve the needs of a population that is already relatively well off at the expense of patients whose needs and expectations of benefit from interventions of the same cost would be greater. Hospice will risk being in the position of competing for funds with more effectively redistributive services, and hospice caregivers will need to decide whether to act in self-interest by lobbying for increased funds or to become effective advocates for increased funding for other pressing Medicare needs, such as increased community support for the elderly living at home and better long-term care arrangements for those who cannot live at home.

Summary and Conclusions

This chapter was written to illuminate the major ethical dilemmas that seem to be facing hospice as a part of the health care system. The fact that ethical dilemmas and problems arise is not a censure — thorny ethical issues are as much a part of life as are death and dying. Nor does the argument above point toward any particular response to hospice or to the new Medicare reimbursement. However, awareness of these issues should lead to increased critical scrutiny of decisions made in response to the exigencies of the moment. Examination of the significance of the issues should also lead to including the consideration of these effects, as policies are established that will determine the future shape of the hospice movement, the character of future hospice workers, and the role of traditional care settings in the care of dying patients.

The focuses of ethical problems that were presented here — the range of treatment options that should be available, informed consent for competent patients, decision making for incompetent patients, and equity in access to care — are ones that confront the entire health care delivery system and the public policies that shape it. As a new component of that system, hospice programs are in a good position to scrutinize their own individual policies and patient care practices as well as the public policies that are beginning to affect them. Hospice's commitment to high-quality, individualized care that reflects the patient's values may be strained by the new legislation that risks compromising individual well-being to serve other societal goals.

Hospices in this country are a new endeavor, one without a substantial definition and traditional role. This can be a weakness if it allows seriously erroneous decisions to be made on these ethical issues. In addition, such errors, if made, are likely to lead to a public outcry that even the best of hospice programs are poorly situated to withstand. The current lack of definition and traditions could prove to be a strength, however, in that hospice providers and others with an interest in hospice can take this rare opportunity to develop a coherent and strong self-definition, enforceable standards of care, and a productive interface with the rest of the health care system.

References

1. Sudnow, D. *Passing On.* Englewood Cliffs, NJ: Prentice-Hall, Inc., 1967.

2. Brim, O. G., and others. *The Dying Patient.* New York: Russell Sage Foundation, 1970.

3. Glaser, B., and Strauss, A. *Awareness of Dying.* Hawthorne, NY: Aldine Publishing Company, 1965.

4. Thomas, L. Dying as failure. *Annals of the American Academy of Political and Social Science.* 1980. 447:1.

5. Zorza, V., and Zorza, R. *A Way to Die.* New York: Alfred A. Knopf, 1980.

6. Zorza and Zorza.

7. Saunders, C. *The Management of Terminal Disease.* London: Edward Arnold, 1978.

8. Millett, N. Hospice: Challenging society's approach to death. *Health and Social Work.* 1979. 4:131.

9. Alsoform, J. The 'hospice' way of dying—at home with friends and family. *American Medical News.* 1977 Feb. 21. pp. 7-9.

10. Zimmerman, J. M. *Hospice: Complete Care for the Terminally Ill.* Baltimore: Urban & Schwarzenberg, 1981.

11. Department of Health, Education, and Welfare. *Facts of Life and Death.* Washington, DC: U.S. Government Printing Office, 1978, pp. 31-33.

12. Saunders, C. Appropriate treatment, appropriate death. In: Saunders, *The Management of Terminal Disease.* pp. 1-18.

13. President's Commission for the Study of Ethical Problems in Medicine and Biomedical and Behavioral Research. *Deciding to Forego Life-Sustaining Treatment.* Washington, DC: U.S. Government Printing Office, 1983.

14. President's Commission. *Deciding to Forego Life-Sustaining Treatment.*

15. Medical treatment decision act. In: *Handbook of Enacted Laws.* New York: Society for the Right to Die, n.d.

16. California Health and Safety Code, Sections 7185-7195, Sacramento, 1976 Sept. 30.

17. The California Natural Death Act: An empirical study of physicians' practices. Note, *Stanford Law Review.* 1979. 31:913.

18. President's Commission. *Deciding to Forego Life-Sustaining Treatment.*

19. Potter, J. F. A challenge for the hospice movement. *New England Journal of Medicine.* 1980. 302:53-55.

20. President's Commission. *Deciding to Forego Life-Sustaining Treatment.*

21. Saunders. *Appropriate Treatment, Appropriate Death.*

22. President's Commission. *Deciding to Forego Life-Sustaining Treatment.*

23. Potter.

24. Lynn, J. Care near the end of life. In: Cassel, C., and Walsh, J. R., editors. *Geriatric Medicine: Principles and Practice.* New York: Springer-Verlag, 1983.

25. Saunders. *Management of Terminal Disease.*

26. Millett.

27. President's Commission. *Deciding to Forego Life-Sustaining Treatment.*

28. Kuzma, A. L. Hospice: The legal ramifications of a place to die. *Indiana Law Journal.* 1981. 56: 673-702.

29. Oakes, G. A. A prosecutor's view of treatment decisions, and Ginex, G. R. A prosecutor's view on liability for withholding or withdrawing medical care: The myth and the reality. In: Doudera, A. E., and Peters, J. D., editors. *Legal and Ethical Aspects of Treating Critically and Terminally Ill Patients.* Ann Arbor, MI: AUPHA Press, 1982.

30. President's Commission. *Deciding to Forego Life-Sustaining Treatment.*

31. Erle, H. Terminal care: The national scene and the individual patient. In: Reidenbert, M., editor. *Clinical Pharmacology of Symptom Control.* Vol. 66, No. 5, *The Medical Clinics of North America.* Philadelphia: W. B. Saunders Co., 1982.

32. Baines, M. J. Control of other symptoms. In: Saunders, *The Management of Terminal Disease.* pp. 102-3.

33. Saunders. *Management of Terminal Disease.*

34. President's Commission. *Deciding to Forego Life-Sustaining Treatment.*

35. President's Commission. *Deciding to Forego Life-Sustaining Treatment.*

36. Kuzma.

37. Oakes.

38. Zerwekh, J. V. The dehydration question. *Nursing 83.* 1983. p. 47.

39. President's Commission. *Deciding to Forego Life-Sustaining Treatment.*

40. Zerwekh.

41. President's Commission for the Study of Ethical Problems in Biomedical and Behavioral Research. *Making Health Care Decisions.* Washington, DC: U.S. Government Printing Office, 1982.

42. The Tax Equity and Fiscal Responsibility Act of 1982, Sec. 122; Public Law 97-248, Congress of the United States.

43. Department of Health and Human Services, Health Care Financing Administration. Draft of a proposed rule, dated 3/17/83, Washington, DC.

44. President's Commission. *Deciding to Forego Life-Sustaining Treatment.*

45. Potter.

46. President's Commission. *Making Health Care Decisions.*

47. President's Commission. *Deciding to Forego Life-Sustaining Treatment.*

48. Lynn, J., and Childress, J. F. Must a patient always be given food and water? *Hastings Center Report.* 1983 Oct. 13(5):17-22.

49. Sacred Congregation for the Doctrine of the Faith. *Declaration on Euthanasia.* The Vatican, 1980 June 26.

50. Sacred Congregation.

51. President's Commission. *Making Health Care Decisions.*

52. Mudd, P. High ideals and hard cases: The evolution of a hospice. *Hastings Center Report.* 1982. 12:11-14.

53. President's Commission. *Making Health Care Decisions.*

54. Tax Equity and Fiscal Responsibility Act.

55. Dept. Health and Human Services, HCFA.

56. President's Commission. *Deciding to Forego Life-Sustaining Treatment.*

57. President's Commission. *Deciding to Forego Life-Sustaining Treatment.*

58. President's Commission. *Deciding to Forego Life-Sustaining Treatment.*

59. California Health and Safety Code.

60. President's Commission for the Study of Ethical Problems in Biomedical and Behavioral Research. *Securing Access to Health Care.* Washington, DC: U.S. Government Printing Office, 1983.

61. President's Commission. *Securing Access to Health Care.*

62. Mudd.

63. Tax Equity and Fiscal Responsibility Act.

64. Dept. Health and Human Services, HCFA.

65. Dept. Health and Human Services, HCFA.

66. Sudnow.

67. Brim and others.

68. Glaser and Strauss.

69. President's Commission. *Securing Access to Health Care.*

70. Osterweis, M., and Champagne, D. S. The U.S. hospice movement: Issues in development. *American Journal of Public Health.* 1979 May. 69:492-96.

71. American Hospital Association. Statement to the House Committee on Ways and Means: H.R. 5180, Coverage of Hospice Care under the Medicare Program. Washington, DC, 1982 March 31.

Chapter 11

Issues in Hospice Administration

Dottie C. Wilson and David J. English, D.P.A.

More than half of the new businesses formed each year in this country fail within the first two years. The primary reason for these failures has been determined to be inadequate, inexperienced management.[1] Hospice programs may fail for the same reason, even though it may seem difficult to visualize hospices as businesses. Generally, hospice staff uphold such a high purpose in tending to the needs of terminally ill patients and their families that people sometimes assume hospices should not be compared with business operations. Experience has shown, however, that hospices are not immune and that they can fail, particularly if the administrative strengths of successful businesses are lacking. We have found that many programs, whose planners and staff have had the best intentions toward patients and families, failed because of insufficient or inadequate developmental and operational management.[2,3] They have suffered from lack of clarity in the allocation of administrative responsibility, from inattention to budgeting or financing, from assumptions of agreement not contractually confirmed, from insufficient emphasis on staff selection and training, and from inadequate communication — not only internally but also externally, with the health care community and the public at large.

This chapter was initially prepared for publication in *The Hospice: Development and Administration,* 2nd edition (in press), edited by Glen W. Davidson and published by Hemisphere Publishing Corporation, copyright 1984. It is reproduced here by permission of the editor and the Hemisphere Publishing Corporation.

It is understandable that hospice administrators have run into difficulties of this sort, especially because the movement itself is so young. Staff at the first hospice program in the United States began care in 1974, and the concept is new to the health care community. Hospice initiators, possessing a wide variety of motivations and skills, have developed a broad range of organizational structures, or models, acceptable to both their own philosophies of hospice care and the specific needs of their communities. We feel that the early hospice initiators were creative, energetic, and zealous in developing their programs. Some created centers of excellence, whereas others struggled in vain. Over the past 10 years, many needed programs have been planned but not introduced. Some hospice staff have been able to implement programs only partially, and some others have begun providing care and then failed This lack of consistent and steady growth has been due primarily to three factors:

- An uninformed public—the transitional lag between initial program development and enthusiastic community support[4-6]
- Externally imposed limitations—financial and regulatory restrictions that threaten economic viability[7-10]
- Internal administrative inadequacy—lack of expertise of some hospice administrators in program planning, implementation, and management[11-13]

As a result, many hospice programs currently in operation consist of a variety of nonintegrated components, partially implemented components, and subcontracted services, which may have considerable diversity of organizational structure and goal emphasis. In addition to this amorphous mass of existing programs, new programs of various designs are being planned by a wide variety of community groups and organizations. Various permutations of these structures have been described as hospice "models," although definitions of models have been neither clear nor standardized.[14-17]

Since it is in terms of models that administrative issues need to be considered, we have chosen to discuss first organizational structure by model and then to address the issues.

Organizational Structure

The designation of models, categories, or other structural groupings of hospice programs seemingly represents a transitional stage in hospice program development that apparently is unique to this country.[18] In this essay, organizational structures of existing hospice programs have been divided into two general groups: independent and dependent hospices. Organizational strengths and problems are outlined for each group.

Independent or Freestanding Hospices

Staff in independent organizations may provide care or may coordinate care provided by others.[19-22] Hospices providing direct care frequently contract for additional services to supplement their own care. Home care is provided and possibly direct inpatient care also in a freestanding facility. (In organizations without an inpatient facility, *home* generally is defined as "where the patient is." This distinction allows "home" visits to patients, whether actually in the home or in a conventional inpatient setting.) It might be helpful to describe four types of the independent hospice model.

The first type is the primarily volunteer organization, which may encompass an entire city or county. Volunteer programs generally have provisions for professional and lay volunteer services. There frequently are some paid administrative staff members who are funded from foundation and individual contributions. Volunteer program developers have sought independence primarily to gain administrative autonomy. Many of these individuals believe that "true" hospice care can be provided only outside the health care system. In general, these programs are grass roots efforts with local community boards and extensive community support. Administrative knowledge and experience, however, have tended to be inadequate—as has support from the medical community.

Problems that characterize independent volunteer programs include staff burnout because of inadequate procedures, policies, and staff support; small bases of referral because of both antagonism from physicians and other health care professionals and lack of quality control; and program failure resulting from inadequate funding or contractual documentation. Eventually, the viability of these volunteer-dominated programs may be limited severely by hospice accreditation requirements. Although some of these organizations have been closed and more will probably be closed in the future, their staffs have performed a valuable service in demonstrating the hospice concept and providing an example of hospice care for others.

A second type of program in this group is the nonvolunteer program—licensed as a home health agency or other formal structure within the health care system—which is being reimbursed for care to the greatest extent possible. These programs are expected to survive and may prosper if their management gives sufficient attention to both quality of patient care and excellence of administration.

A third type of program is the coordinating organization. These programs do not provide direct care; rather, they frequently consist of small administrative groups that contract all direct care to home health agencies and hospitals. Administrators themselves provide coordination, trained volunteers, training to the contracted staff, and public education (some of the nonreimbursable hospice activities).

In a coordinating organization, a single program may encompass the entire community. As in the first type of independent model, because most of these programs are grass roots efforts, administrative expertise frequently is inadequate. Administrative problems include inadequate quality of care and contracts that may be incomplete or not legally binding. Contracted staff may not be designated as hospice staff and in fact may allocate only a small percentage of their time to hospice work. The result can be low quality hospice care.

Another major difficulty in this type of organization is ensuring continuity of care among several contracted organizations, no one of which is really "in charge" of the patient's care. Mammoth administrative and educational efforts are required by program staff to ensure both high quality and continuity of care. Without such efforts, hospice failure, staff burnout, and inappropriate care frequently result. For these reasons, high-quality hospice care cannot be expected from programs that contract all of their direct patient care. These programs, however, appear to be transitional organizations that may meld into more stable structures as reimbursement mechanisms for hospice care improve and hospice accreditation is established.

A fourth type of independent program may be identified by its advocates: the independent program not providing care, not contracting care, but supplying volunteer "friendly visitors" and "patient advocates." The National Hospice Organization has defined hospice as "a program of palliative and supportive services which provides physical, psychological, social and spiritual care for dying persons and their families. Services are provided by a medically supervised interdisciplinary team of professionals and volunteers"[23] Although this fourth type of program may be helpful in the absence of a hospice, it should be clarified that it is not a hospice according to the above definition.

Dependent Hospices

These programs have been formed as a part of one or more larger organizations: a hospital, skilled nursing facility, home health agency or consortium.[24-28] Some hospitals with hospice programs have home care departments. Others frequently offer contracted services for care not supplied directly. Most employ designated hospice staff for all services provided in most dependent programs. Frequently, staff members work full time for the hospice. There may be no full-time designated staff, however, or there may be a combination of both full-time and part-time staff.

In this structure, administrative strengths and problems can be identified more clearly. Strengths include the administrative expertise and financial stability of the parent organization and a large physician referral base, since the program operates within the established health care system. If the parent organization is a large hospital, additional strengths include the availability of an interdisciplinary breadth of personnel and already established training and support systems. Problems that occur in dependent hospice programs include loss of autonomy, the discouraging factor that patients unable to pay might not be admitted, and a tendency toward more conventional care rather than specialized hospice care.

The motivations of hospitals, nursing homes, and home health agencies in introducing hospice programs may be quite different from those of independent hospices. Program goals of trying to fill beds, compete with other institutions, increase the number of home care visits, and produce other (primarily financial) gains are often at odds with the hospice concept. These programs may fail or accreditation may be denied — in spite of administrative adequacy — if team function, high quality of care, and high quality of life for patients and families are not primary objectives.

In order to survive and succeed, all hospice staff need to provide both high-quality care and high-quality administrative organization and function. Stressing the importance of integrating good care with administration, John E. Fryer states that the "very best treatment intentions will not be carried out if administrative skill is absent. The best administrative scheme is of no value without the proper motivating force."[29]

In this essay, rather than attempting an exhaustive examination of administrative issues for the developmental stages of each hospice model, we have outlined the major administrative issues relevant to all hospice managements, whether providing or planning care. These issues are presented from a background of experience in administration, business, and other areas of health care, as well as in hospice management. Viewed from the perspective of our years of experience in assisting hospices nationwide in planning, developing, financing, and managing their programs, these issues are basic to the long-term success of any hospice program.

Administrative Issues

Seven major administrative issues for hospices are outlined in this section: structure and function, finance, professional assistance, public relations, patient and family care, personnel, and evaluation and research. Each of these issues needs to be addressed, to the best of ability and resources, by administrators of every hospice program — regardless of structure.

Issues Relative to Structure and Function

The administrative structure and function of hospice programs have a significant effect on their stability and success. Because dependent and independent programs are structurally distinct, this issue is considered separately for each of these groups.

Independent Hospices

Independent hospice organizations that form their own corporate entities are well advised to examine the following structural aspects:

Incorporation. The documents of incorporation need to be prepared by an attorney skilled in such work. A lawyer who is a member of the program's founding board may prove particularly helpful.

Bylaws. The bylaws of the corporation should be no more restrictive than is legally necessary. In writing the bylaws, planners should allow for programmatic expansion and organizational growth. They should also ensure that no one official can control program development. The procedure for changing or adding bylaws should be specified.

The appointment of officials and directors (or trustees), the frequency of meetings of the board of directors, and the quorum required for meetings should be specified in the bylaws. Officials usually include a chairman, one or more vice-chairmen, a secretary, and a treasurer. Meetings of the board of directors often are needed monthly in the hospice's early development, with a simple procedure stated for calling special meetings to deal with special problems that develop in the interim between legally required meetings. Once the program is fully operational, board meetings may be held less frequently. The quorum for board meetings needs to be carefully considered — it should be large enough for responsible decision making yet not so large that it is difficult to obtain. One well-known hospice organization had several board resignations at one time, thus making a legal quorum impossible.

Board of Directors. The size and composition of the board of directors is important. The board should include the number of people needed to accomplish its purposes and still not be so large as to be unwieldy. In some programs a large influential board and a small executive committee are established, with the recognition that few of the community leaders on the board will attend monthly meetings. The executive committee meets frequently and becomes the decision-making body.

In other programs the number of board members is kept to a minimum, but these members are very active. Influential citizens are invited to become members of an advisory committee to the board. This latter structural decision allows the influence of community leaders to be utilized for the benefit of the hospice, but confines the decision-making board to a small, knowledgeable, participatory nucleus. The obvious advantages of this latter organizational structure seem to make it more effective than the former and certainly more effective than a large board with no executive committee.

All boards tend to go through two stages: the founding board and the operating board. The members of the founding board are the program's initiators and frequently include its future supervisory personnel. Once the program is planned and established, however, new talents usually are needed for its ongoing operation and growth. Some founding board members then need to step aside—moving on to either hospice staff functions or new initiatives elsewhere. Once this decision has been made, additional operating board members should be installed. Key members of the operating board need to be practical and successful businessmen sympathetic to the hospice concept. They should be acquainted with each other and meet informally in their normal business activities, not only at hospice board meetings. Bankers, accountants, attorneys, private businessmen, former directors of foundations, religious leaders, cancer center directors, or directors of other health care institutions are likely candidates. It may be helpful to install citizens who are serving concurrent terms as members of boards of charitable or other health care organizations. Successful business and community leaders can contribute significantly to the financial viability and stability of the hospice.

A word of caution is in order concerning the relationship between staff and board members. No staff members should be voting members. No staff other than the executive director and perhaps the medical director should attend board meetings, except to provide special education or reports. Difficulties may arise for staff members who were formerly members of a founding board and were accustomed to participating in policy decision making. It may be necessary to clarify to staff that the purpose of the board is to set policy and that of the staff is to implement policy. Communicating this same information to the board is often necessary.

Leadership. The leadership and operational management of the hospice is in the hands of the executive director (or administrator or program coordinator) and the medical director. Because of the importance of the executive director's administrative expertise in independent programs, the medical director seldom has the experience to fill this position successfully. The position of medical director needs to be filled by an experienced, respected, and dedicated licensed physician. One potential problem may be alleviated if planners recognize that choosing as medical director the community's leading oncologist, for example, necessitates giving attention to developing a broader referral base—and not depending on the medical director's referrals alone.

Dependent Hospices

The status of a hospice in the organizational structure of a particular institution is evidence of the degree to which that institution is committed to the hospice concept. Administrative planners for a dependent hospice within a hospital need to ensure that the program has sufficient organizational status to be viable and to maintain program autonomy.

Governance. Because patients in a hospital-based hospice are drawn from a number of clinical departments (including medicine, surgery, oncology, and gynecology), and resources are drawn from other departments (such as social service, physical therapy, chaplaincy, and dietary units), the dependent hospice needs to be at least at the same level in the organizational structure as other major departments within the institution. In our experience, programs established as part of an oncology or nursing department have had major difficulties in both viability and program autonomy.

Space. Dependent hospice staff can provide high-quality care and develop interdisciplinary team care most successfully when housed in a separate inpatient unit. It is important to negotiate with the institution early in the development process. If this is not done, the hospice program may be interpreted by some groups within the institution as a threat to their own financial viability. The size of the hospice unit should be based on carefully gathered statistical information so that a high occupancy rate may be achieved. Otherwise the institution's revenue may be reduced or heads of other departments may attempt to fill hospice beds with non-hospice patients.

Budget. The hospice should be self-sufficient and not wholly dependent on the institution for funding. In addition to third-party payments and patient-generated revenues, hospice administrators should develop local funding sources.

Leadership. With the hospice at the departmental level, the hospice directorship holds a position of power within the institution. This position in a dependent hospice has been filled most successfully by a respected physician with administrative expertise. Such an individual is able to foster high-quality patient care in the hospice and to educate the rest of the institution staff in the hospice concept. In addition, the hospice director can ensure the financial viability of the program and carry out administrative management tasks. As is the case with independent hospices, the hospice director needs to develop a broad referral base and not depend solely on personal referrals to the program.

Staffing Autonomy. Hospice managers need to have the power to recruit and employ their own staff at a status comparable to that of other departments within the institution. Experience has shown that higher quality staff are attracted if hospice administrators perform their own recruitment and screening. Institutional resources, including the personnel department, naturally should be utilized when of benefit to the hospice.

Because the staff-patient ratio needs to be higher in an inpatient unit than on regular medical or surgical floors, hospice planners should obtain a written agreement with the institution that this ratio will be maintained regardless of staff shortages elsewhere in the hospital. This agreement should be obtained prior to the opening of the hospice unit.

Development Time. The leadership of both the hospice and its umbrella institution needs to dedicate sufficient time to develop this program. It may take a number of years and considerable financial outlay to educate decision makers and to plan and negotiate program details. Once established, hospice management needs to devote additional time to cementing relationships, building interdisciplinary teams, improving patient and family care, and stimulating financial and program growth.

Comparison of Independent and Dependent Hospices

Differences in structure and function between independent and dependent hospices have evolved in such a way so as to clarify the strengths and weaknesses of each. A comparison of the administrative encumbrances relative to each may be helpful.

Administrators of independent hospices report to the board of directors and carry out its policies but also may be able to influence those policies. They have considerable autonomy but no power. Although they have control over their operating budgets, these administrators have to work with only limited financial resources. They tend to develop strong community linkages but have to put more effort into obtaining needed services and support systems.

Administrators of dependent hospices more often have resources and support from the larger organization but tend to lack community linkages. Although a part of the seat of power, they have the disadvantage of being accountable to it. Such administrators lack control over their own budgets and policies. Their activities are in coordination and internal politics.

Other researchers working independently have noted the dichotomy between independent and dependent hospices. In 1982, for example, Robert W. Buckingham and Dale Lupu commented on the emergence of

> two divergent types of hospice programs: independent, heavily volunteer hospices with a variety of professional staff delivering a wide array of social/psychological services to the home but having major funding problems; and institutionally based hospices providing inpatient care, more medical/nursing services, fewer social/psychological services and having fewer types of volunteers and staff. Institutionally based hospices reported 50 percent fewer funding problems, implying that a major advantage of institutional affiliation is financial support.[30]

Issues Relative to Finances

The many important administrative issues relative to finances are considered together for both dependent and independent hospices under the following headings: financial viability, reimbursement, other funding, and financial management.

Financial Viability

The financial viability of a hospice program depends on its corporate structure, the service components included in its program, and its ability both to maximize reimbursement and to obtain additional funds to cover non-reimbursable costs. The legislation that makes hospice a covered service under the Medicare program[31] is an important positive addition but should not be viewed as the solution to all of hospice's financial problems.

If the corporate structure is that of an independent hospice, and reimbursement is received for the care provided, financial viability depends on covering the organization's overhead costs. This is a function of program size, which, in turn, is dependent upon several factors: the population of the geographic area served, the hospice-eligible patient pool, and the referral pattern. Administrators for an independent hospice home health agency serving solely hospice patients may find it impossible to operate efficiently and effectively over a long period of time if the population served is less than half a million.

When the program includes an independent inpatient facility, the reimbursement rate is a key factor: if the reimbursement rate is at the skilled nursing facility level, a significant discrepancy may exist between cost and reimbursement, particularly for Medicaid-eligible patients. Reimbursement may range from $30 to $100 per inpatient day, for example, whereas actual cost may exceed $200 per inpatient day.

Although the costs of patient care in programs contractually affiliated with other organizations may be covered by the reimbursement structures of the affiliated organizations, the separate hospice administrative costs remain a problem. These costs are unlikely to be recoverable as overhead, particularly if the affiliated organization is a home health agency whose overhead costs already exceed the Medicare maximum. In such programs, additional funds often must be sought to cover these costs.

When the hospice is part of another organization, financial viability is ensured more easily because overhead can be spread over the broader patient load of the entire organization. In addition, some part-time or consultant staff may be allocated from the larger organization to the hospice unit without additional overall cost. Such staff may include chaplains, pharmacists, dietitians, and therapists.

The service components included in the hospice program affect the program's reimbursement level and thus its financial viability. A fully occupied inpatient hospice unit in an acute care facility may be entirely reimbursable, whereas even with the new regulation, only a small part of bereavement follow-up service is reimbursable. With the education component of the hospice program, in-service education of reimbursable patient care staff is covered, but other professional, volunteer, and public education costs are not easily reimbursable because these costs frequently fall outside those considered necessary and prudent.

Reimbursement

Maximizing reimbursement can become a highly developed skill in hospice administration. Such an endeavor includes careful record keeping of all reimbursable activities by all staff, selection of the most helpful fiscal intermediary (if a choice is available), negotiation with the appropriate review organizations to develop proper inpatient admission guidelines, and reliance on lay and professional volunteers to perform nonreimbursable services. In addition, maximizing reimbursement means paying close attention to the details of the regulations. Services that are reimbursable, for instance, if performed by a home health aide but not if performed by a nurse should always be performed by a home health aide. If the hospice program and the patient are operating under the 1982 Medicare changes, these shifts in care provider may not be necessary. Demonstration projects, particularly with Blue Cross-Blue Shield, continue to be negotiated by a number of program administrators for increased reimbursement over a short term (usually one or two years).

Other Funding

Virtually all hospice programs need other funding in addition to reimbursements to cover costs, although the percentage of costs to be covered through such funds varies with the factors described earlier. The key to success in fund-raising is to develop a comprehensive funding strategy. This means a strategy cutting across a broad range of available sources and not dependent upon only one source. Possible sources include:
- Federal, state, and county governments
- Foundations
- Corporations, associations, unions
- Private individuals
- Special interest groups
- General public

As most funding sources require competitive applications, hospice administrators need to possess or develop grant writing skills. In applying to funding sources, the funding strategy must ensure that the right source is contacted by the right individuals with the right message at the right time and place. Some hospice administrators have learned this by bitter experience. In one program, large individual donations were received before the hospice had been granted 501C(3) status to accept tax deductible donations. Program planners for another hospice began their fund-raising drive three days after a major United Way drive was launched. In one community, administrators of two competing programs approached the same funding source at the same time, were openly critical of each other, and were both rejected.[32]

Financial Management

Financial management in all its aspects is the responsibility of the hospice administration. Accurate and complete financial record keeping is essential. In our experience, nevertheless, the accounting tool omitted most frequently by hospice administrators is the cash flow projection. Independent hospices have been found to have a particularly low level of sophistication in accounting and finance, yet they are the ones with the greatest financial problems. In fact, one program was discovered to maintain no financial records — not even a list of memorial donations.

At a minimum, each hospice administration needs to keep the following accurate and up-to-date financial records:

- Cash receipts and disbursements journal
- General ledger
- Financial statements (prepared monthly by an internal bookkeeper)
- Budget for the next twelve months
- Cash flow projections

Financial management means many other responsibilities as well: collecting receivable accounts and promised donations, banking, paying bills without duplicating payments, issuing correctly prepared checks (one program staffer issued checks with one signature instead of the required two, and another inappropriately used a rubber stamp for the second signature), and ensuring that there are sufficient funds to cover the checks written. Similarly, payments to the government for deductions at source need to be issued on time, with proper documentation and reports.

Administrators must also ensure that the board does not become liable because of any financial actions or inactions of the program management. This admonition is pertinent to boards of both community-based independent programs and major institutions.

Issues Relative to Professional Assistance

Issues that deal with professional assistance and agreements in hospice operation and development are discussed under the following headings: legal counsel, accounting, insurance, quality of care review, consulting, and agreements and contracts.

Legal Counsel

All hospice programs at one time or another are in need of legal assistance and advice. If a board of directors wants to take an action, for example, it needs to know its legal liability. Contracts and agreements between the hospice program and other organizations need legal review. Many hospice programs have an attorney as a member of the board of directors. This attorney can advise the board as to when legal assistance is appropriate and perhaps may provide it at no charge. (Note: Be careful. Sometimes you get what you pay for!)

Accounting

Hospice administrators (or those administrators in the organization of which the hospice is a part) should obtain professional accounting assistance in developing their financial books and records, establishing charts of accounts, preparing annual financial statements, and completing Form 990 income tax reports. Independent incorporated hospice programs should have an annual financial audit performed.

Insurance

There are a number of different kinds of insurance coverage necessary in order to protect hospice programs against a variety of risks. Needed insurance coverage includes both worker's compensation and medical malpractice, liability, property, and automobile insurance. A federal requirement for all paid staff, worker's compensation covers employees in the event of injury while on the job. Malpractice insurance should be obtained for all individuals visiting patients, both staff members and volunteers. Liability insurance is needed to cover paid staff members, lay volunteers, and board members. Automobile insurance protects the organization against lawsuits in the event of staff members being involved in automobile accidents while on hospice business. Although this insurance does not cover damage to a staff vehicle, it does protect the corporation should an accident result in a suit for damages. Health insurance as a staff fringe benefit should be considered, as well as the proportion of such insurance to be paid through the hospice program.

Finally, bonding may be desirable to cover staff while visiting patients' homes in order to protect the corporation against claims of theft. Unfortunately, bonding is very expensive and may be difficult to obtain. As an alternative, some hospice administrators have developed elaborate procedures for volunteers in the home so as to minimize the potential risk of suits from patients or family members. Care must be taken not to let these procedures become so cumbersome that they affect the quality of services delivered.

Quality of Care Review

Internal audits should be performed on a regular basis to ensure a high quality of medical and nursing care. Rehabilitation audits may also be possible, although the criteria and standards tend to be more difficult to define and apply than those for medical and nursing care.

Consulting

Many hospice administrators have found themselves turning to consulting firms with seemingly unsolvable dilemmas. Unfortunately, many administrators, particularly those of the independent hospice programs, may have little understanding of how, where, and when to utilize consulting firms.

A formal agreement between the hospice administrator and the consulting firm should specify the expectations of the hospice program, the specific scope of work, the time frame for its accomplishment, and the price involved. This contract or agreement should be made available for review by all appropriate staff so that the scope of work is mutually understood. Significant tension developed in one hospice program when the board of directors, which had unanimously approved a consulting contract, had not convinced the staff of the value of this financial commitment.

Consulting firms are used most effectively when there is a need for their specific expertise in areas such as reimbursement, fund raising, program development, and administrative issues. Probably the single most important role that a consultant can play is that of an outside facilitator of change within the organization. It is not uncommon for consultants to relay to board and staff information that they already know; however, because it comes from an outside "expert," this information has some additional credibility.

Hospice administrators should always obtain fixed-price contracts with a specific scope of work and a specific time frame. Consultants who offer an open-ended contract to provide open-ended services should be avoided.

Agreements and Contracts

Verbal understandings and agreements are important first steps, but they must be put in writing and signed by all parties. Many hospice staff members, believing that written agreements show a lack of faith in other parties involved, are reluctant to enter into written contracts and letters of agreement. This reluctance may be responsible later for destroying harmony among the concerned parties. All significant agreements and understandings should be expressed in writing, to inform all parties—both present and future—as to the specific understandings made. With written form, both parties are forced to be more precise as to what has been agreed.

A letter of agreement may be the natural forerunner of a legal contract, particularly for inpatient institutions for which it is necessary to contract for home care services with a home health agency. All of the details of the agreement should be specified in the letter, and it should be signed by both parties. Many letters of agreement are unenforceable or too costly to enforce; therefore, they are useful only in providing documentation of respective organizational positions and agreements. Legal contractual agreements should be prepared to cover contracted care, inpatient units, purchase of equipment, employment agreements with staff, and all other relevant formal arrangements with others.

Issues Relative to Public Relations

It is important to allocate time for public relations planning and execution both at the initial stages and on a continuing basis so that the program can gain widespread recognition and long-term success. Public relations is essential in a number of significant hospice areas.

Interorganizational Liaison

Generally, hospice goals include meeting the physical, psychosocial, and spiritual needs of patients and their families, providing inpatient care, home care, bereavement care, and continuity of care — and including education and research as program components. The interdisciplinary nature of hospice care demands that close attention be paid to relationships between the hospice program itself and the many community organizations involved. These organizations may include: those providing direct patient care; community resources supplying ancillary services such as equipment or meals; support services such as mental health services, churches and volunteer groups; financial organizations (including government and private insurance offices); licensing bureaus; and education and research institutions (primarily universities). Continuing good relations with these multiple organizations are essential to their cooperation with and support of the hospice program.

Medical Community Involvement

Physicians and physician organizations such as local medical societies need to be involved in the hospice program from the time of its initial planning onward.[33] Patient care must be directed by physicians. Broad physician support is essential to maximize ongoing patient referrals to the program. Indeed, the percentage of hospice-eligible patient referrals is usually in direct proportion to the level of physician support. This support is acquired and nurtured over time, not only through education but also through demonstrating the need for hospice and the quality of care provided. Independent program staff outside the health care system frequently appear antagonistic to the system and to physicians, to their own detriment. If they have not sought physician involvement early in their planning, these individuals have suffered unnecessarily throughout their program's often short-lived existence. Hospice administrators should seek common ground with local physicians and gradually develop physician involvement and support.

General Public Support

Public education has been a function of most hospice programs, particularly the independent ones. Indeed, education has been cited in the literature as the fourth component of a hospice program. Yet, in spite of the work of Elisabeth Kübler-Ross and those who followed, many people in this country are still not familiar with the concept or how it may be actualized.[34-38] Public education needs ongoing attention by hospice administrators. The benefits of public education should be obvious: referrals, donations, volunteers, and public support of hospice-enabling legislation.

Public relations for community support may be conducted in numerous ways, all of which are time-consuming but not necessarily expensive.[39-41] Included in these public relations endeavors are:

Lectures. Talks by physicians or other hospice staff or by volunteers, sometimes through a speakers' bureau, are the basic sources of community support. These may be informal talks to small church or club groups, lectures to professionals or students, major addresses in public forums, or radio or television interviews. As there is a continuing drain on personnel providing these talks, each request must be reported and then considered in terms of the balance between staff availability and program benefits. The use of slides, films, and other teaching materials contributes to the success of these activities.

Written Materials. Utilization of these materials is a time-honored method for contributing to public education and eliciting support. Written materials may include articles for publication in magazines or journals, brochures describing the hospice program, and newsletters. Although newsletters require regular preparation and the development and maintenance of a mailing list, they are useful in disseminating both general educational information and information about program progress and needs. The outlay of funds for printing and mailing is necessary, but donations frequently can help defray these costs.

Media-generated Materials. Reporters and other nonhospice personnel can be encouraged to produce material for newspapers, magazines, radio, television, and films. The hospice, as a new and compelling concept, tends to be of great interest to the media. Because this interest may be sincere and altruistic, it usually is welcomed by hospice program developers. Enthusiasm should be tempered with caution, however, so that media coverage does not "backfire" or have a detrimental effect on the program or its patients. Firm control is essential to ensure that the coverage is accurate, timely, and nonthreatening (to potential patients, families, physicians, funding sources, and others). Careful timing is necessary to prevent major coverage before the program is ready so as to avoid premature referrals and consequent disappointments. Timing the coverage to coincide with the opening of new services or with fund-raising campaigns tends to be most productive. It is difficult to maintain a level of control over what will be delivered to the public because reporters frequently do not agree to a review of their work before publication. They may even seek unofficial (and often less accurate) sources of information. Good public relations contacts with local media management as well as careful education of reporters can do much to ensure both timing and control of media coverage.

Issues Relative to Patient and Family Care

Hospice planners and administrators are responsible for developing policies, criteria, and procedures for patient and family care. They may benefit from the expertise of others in this task—not only from staff and community experts but also from the experience of other hospice programs and from available literature. Methods need to be developed to ensure that policies and procedures are followed and can be modified as necessary. The following areas are essential for decision making.

Patient Pool/Patient Load

To plan the program's size, organization, and staffing, it is necessary to determine not only which services will be provided (such as home care, inpatient care, bereavement follow-up, day care, and outpatient care) and the timing of the introduction of each but also the size of the patient pool.[42, 43] Decisions need to be made concerning the catchment area for each service component and the diagnoses acceptable. These decisions must take into account the proportion of patients with these diagnoses who died over the past few years in the defined catchment area. From this information, the patient load may be determined, based on the anticipated physician referral pattern for these diseases in the area. The experience of similar programs may also be helpful.

Criteria for Admission and Discharge

The criteria for admission and the patient load are closely interrelated. Until some criteria are established, the patient load cannot be determined. All criteria need to be consistent, publicly available, and acceptable not only to staff but also to referral sources and reimbursement agencies. Priorities for admission should also be incorporated, to be utilized when more patients are referred and eligible than can be admitted. A statement of criteria for admission should include all or some of the following:

- The disease of the patient is specified as progressive and causing death. The diseases accepted are listed. If limited to cancer, this limitation should be stated explicitly.
- The stage of the patient's disease and its status as terminal are identified, and the method of determination is stated.
- There is a need for hospice services (such as pain control), and the evidence for such need is documented.
- The availability of hospice staff to care for the patient is stated as a requirement. (The priorities noted above are stated here.)

- The role of the referring physician is identified, such as a requirement for approval of the admission and continued direction of the patient's care.
- A limited prognosis may be required. The prognosis may be stated specifically or generally.
- A statement may be included concerning patient and/or family agreement to the admission.
- An acceptable age of the patient may be indicated when the expertise of the staff is limited, such as a minimum or maximum age requirement.
- The catchment area is specified for home care and may or may not be a criterion for other service components.
- If the presence of a primary caregiver in the home is a program requirement, such a limitation is stated. This situation also may depend on the patient's condition and needs.
- It may be advisable to specify certain limits on patient eligibility for the program's future protection (which may or may not be enforced). For example, patients may be deemed ineligible if they are comatose, if their prognosis extends no further than two days, or in the event that a language barrier does not permit communication with staff.
- A statement may be made that there is to be no discrimination due to race, color, religion, sex, national origin, ability to pay, and so forth.[44-46]

Criteria for discharge also need to be identified and stated. Other than patient death, these criteria may include inappropriate admission and transfer to other facilities or locations outside the hospice's catchment area or care capability. The responsibility for decision making for both admission and discharge also needs to be specified.

Standards of Care

Although conceptual statements such as "caring about" as well as "caring for" patients and families may be helpful, specific standards need to be established by hospice administrators—with the assistance of others. In this way program and training goals can be clarified and program evaluation facilitated.[47-50] The National Hospice Organization's standards of care[51] may be accepted verbatim or may be modified or supplemented by hospice planners. The methodology for ensuring continuity of care needs to be spelled out in the statement of standards.

Care Provision

Hospice administrators are charged with responsibilities in the area of care provision, both to facilitate care delivery and to ensure proper approaches to care through policy statements, training, etc. Humane care, attention to detail in direct patient care, and interdisciplinary approaches to care should be emphasized in administrative directives. Facilitating the delivery of high-quality care means administrators being able and willing to meet with patient care staff and contribute creative solutions or approaches to difficult patient and family problems. Administrators also are responsible for ensuring the availability (frequently through cooperative agreements) of materials, supplies, equipment, transportation, and supplementary services so that the needed care can be provided smoothly and efficiently.

Charting and Reporting

It is the responsibility of hospice administrators — with assistance — to determine the method of charting, the items to be included in the charting, the design and supply of forms, and the procedures for completing them and distributing the copies.

The information needed for reports also must be determined. This latter requirement applies to internal reports such as those related to patient care and evaluation, as well as to external reports designed to meet requirements of funding and regulatory agencies and of public relations.

In addition, the methods for collecting information and the procedures for preparing and submitting reports need to be established. It is often helpful to design reporting systems with quality assurance reviews in mind.

Past administrative experience and, in particular, past health care experience are essential for the successful development of clear, complete charting and reports. Care should be taken that both of these activities are accomplished without excessive burden on patient care staff and at the least possible ongoing administrative cost.

Issues Relative to Personnel

Hospices, like many other organizations, are dependent on their personnel for success and continued existence. Staff selection, training, policies, procedures, and support are all major areas of administrative decision making that have a significant impact on program accomplishments as well as on financial needs. Although much could be written about hospice experience in these areas, the checklist that follows may suffice for experienced administrators.

Personnel Policies and Procedures

Policies and procedures, and the methods for modifying them as necessary, are the responsibility of administrators. These include determination of a number of different points.

Clear Lines of Authority. Organizational charts and supervisory structure should have a clear delineation of the lines of authority. at the same time the customary "role blurring" of hospice care should be maintained.

Job Descriptions. All staff, including supervisors, administrators, and volunteers, need specific job descriptions. These descriptions should include the specific qualifications needed for each position, the place of the position in the supervisory structure, the duties and responsibilities involved, and the support and growth opportunities offered.

Staffing Patterns. Interdisciplinary team operation and ratios of staff to patient are essential—both overall and for each service component.[52,53]

Salaries, Wages, and Fringe Benefits. Although in a few hospice programs nursing staff members are paid by the hour, most are paid a salary. Salary levels vary with community practice, but tend not to be higher than average. Fringe benefits vary from the legal minimum to generous. Ultimately, a balance must be achieved between the ability to attract the appropriate staff and the finances available. Salary problems may arise when the work of regular hospice staff is supplemented by home health agencies or personnel from other institutions, particularly when the variations in salary ranges between these organizations are known to team members. Hospice administrators may need to supplement some of these salaries to reduce staff anxiety and turnover.

Hours of Work. Because of the frequently stressful nature of hospice work, variations in hours of work for direct caregivers and extra time allowances for special leave when stress becomes extreme have been tried. Although no overall rule can be applied as yet, administrative attention does need to be directed to this policy, with some latitude provided.

Recruitment and Selection. Criteria for selection of staff and volunteers should be developed by hospice administrators, who need to state clearly the characteristics or qualifications required of all staff and volunteers. The available literature on hospice care is helpful in this endeavor.[54-58] Given these criteria, recruitment and selection procedures should follow those of good business practice everywhere.[59] Volunteer selection should be performed according to the same stringent procedures, regardless of the fact that volunteer services are provided without financial compensation.

Performance Review. A program of regular staff assessment should be instituted, with forms, procedures and time schedules established. Staff improvement needs identified during this process may have an impact on future staff training and may lead to modifications in the selection criteria.

Staff and Volunteer Education and Support

Since few potential staff have had either training or experience specific to hospice programs, administrators need to provide more educational time and resources than do those in conventional health care organizations. Staff support, a necessary hospice element, may be addressed not only through specific support systems but also through educational activities.[60,61] Administrators should provide at least five distinct program elements: orientation, ongoing in-service education, teaching and learning resources, specific support systems, and outside training.

Orientation. Staff and volunteer orientation should include an introduction to the program and its policies and procedures and also to the hospice concept.

Ongoing In-service Education. Particularly in such a new field, ongoing in-service education is an important program element. With the added benefit of contributing to staff support, continuing education need not be extremely time-consuming; however, it should be scheduled regularly.

Teaching and Learning Resources. A library should be established, a simple record-keeping system instituted, and materials accumulated. Such a library, which may include books, journals, reprints, tapes, and films, can serve a number of functions. It is a resource for staff teaching and learning, research, public relations presentations, and articles.

Specific Support Systems. Staff support systems usually include regularly scheduled support meetings for all direct patient care staff, volunteers, and perhaps administrative staff, facilitated by a psychiatrist, or counselor. Other support systems include staff support persons (frequently physicians, social workers, and chaplains), special leave, and staff parties or other social events. Support systems are intended to provide an outlet for expressions of stress in a supportive environment, an opportunity for team building and respite in times of crisis.

Outside Training. Policies need to be set and resources allocated for outside training of staff. Examples of outside training are relevant courses in local universities or schools, special hospice training courses offered by certain established hospice programs and some private organizations with hospice expertise (as well as those provided by the National Hospice Organization), and conferences and seminars on hospice or related topics sponsored by universities or national associations.

Frequently, the attendance of one staff member at an outside training function enables all staff to learn something of benefit to themselves and to the program.

Issues Relative to Evaluation and Research

A complete hospice program includes professionally conducted evaluation and research. Staff members need to be convinced of the importance of this activity, particularly when difficulties arise in team function because of high staff stress levels.

Program Evaluation

There are four major reasons why hospice administrators should conduct evaluations:

- Most funding sources require a built-in evaluation system when the funds are requested.

- Documentation of evaluation is necessary for reimbursement.
- The quality of care being provided in the hospice is determined formally through evaluation.
- Evaluation affects survival. If hospice administrators have a well-documented positive evaluation of the quality of their program's care, they can assure the board of directors (or those of the larger organization) of benefits of the program.[62-64]

The effectiveness of patient care, staff function, and the impact or potential impact of the program on the medical community, the institutional community, and the general public should be covered in this evaluation. It is the role of hospice administrators to facilitate this evaluation, promote it, and make resources available for its completion. A comprehensive and thorough evaluation requires a well-planned program: hospice planners must have established clear goals and measurable objectives in order to determine whether they are being reached.

Research

The priority assigned to research has a significant impact on the hospice, both on the care it provides and on its reputation. Both the financial decision makers and staff need to recognize the importance of research to the program, because it is only through research that the quality of terminal care can be advanced.

Research methodology should be stringent and replicable. It should have both test and control groups and be as rigorous as clinical trials being performed elsewhere throughout the United States. Considerable assistance may be obtained for research. Research committees, utilizing local university researchers or others skilled in methodology and statistical analysis, can assist in collecting the data.

There is a continuing flow of research and evaluation results in the literature of both the Palliative Care Service in Montreal and the British hospices. This country has lagged behind, with only a few programs performing sophisticated research. As the hospice movement in the United States emerges, it is important that American contributions to the art of hospice care be produced and published.

Conclusion

Administrators play an important role in virtually all aspects of hospice planning, implementation, and management. They largely determine policy making, financing, public relations, and evaluation and play supportive roles in problem-solving and facilitating program growth, patient and family care, staff selection, and staff education. Administrators are the representatives of their programs to regulatory and funding agencies and, frequently, to the community as well. In order to fulfill these responsibilities, these individuals should be knowledgeable both about health care administration in general and about their own hospice programs in particular. In addition, they should possess the motivations and characteristics common to all dedicated hospice personnel.

The existing body of experience and knowledge in hospice administration offers direction if not clear guidelines for hospice programs. In all hospice policy and program areas, there is little place today for the trial and error method, the "we'll develop our own" approach or the "n.i.h." (not invented here) syndrome. Administrative management skills in hospices need not be reinvented. Thus, it behooves hospice initiators and planners to be thoroughly familiar with the literature and heed the advice of others. In this way, they will be able to safeguard their programs' survival and stimulate growth through appropriate attention to administrative issues in both planning and operational management.

References

1. Fix, A. J., and Daughton, D. You can bet on it. *Inc.* 1980 December. p. 52.

2. English, D. J., and Wilson, D. C. *The development of guidelines for the HSA review and planning of hospice programs.* (A report prepared for the Health Systems Agency of Southeastern Pennsylvania in Philadelphia). Bethesda, MD: ELM Services, Inc., 1979 May.

3. English, D. J., and Wilson, D. C. Steps in the development of a hospice program. In: *Supplement to Delegate Manual: Association of Community Cancer Centers, 1978.* Bethesda, MD: ELM Services, Inc., revised 1979.

4. Koff, T. H. *Hospice: A Caring Community.* Cambridge, MA: Winthrop Publishers, Inc., 1980.

5. Osterweis, M., and Champagne, D. S. The U.S. hospice movement: Issues in development. *American Journal of Public Health.* 1979. 69(5):492-96.

6. Wilson, D. C. How to obtain community support. In: *The "How To" of Hospice Care* (Report of the Third National Hospice Symposium). Kentfield, CA: Hospice of Marin, 1977. pp. 30-36.

7. National Hospice Organization. *Delivery and payment of hospice services: Investigative study, final report, September, 1979.* McLean, VA: NHO, 1979.

8. English, D. J. The "how to" of evaluation. In: *The "How To" of Hospice Care* (Report of the Third National Hospice Symposium). Kentfield, CA: Hospice of Marin, 1977. pp. 37-41.

9. General Accounting Office. *Report to the Congress: Hospice Care — A Growing Concept in the United States* (HRD-79-50). Washington, DC: U.S. Government Printing Office, 1979.

10. Hackley, J. A. Financing and accrediting hospices. *Hospital Progress.* 1979 March. pp. 51-53.

11. General Accounting Office.

12. Breindel, C. L., and Boyle, R. M. Implementing a multiphased hospice program. *Hospital Progress.* 1979 March. pp. 42-45.

13. Wilson, D. C., English, D. J., and Research Staff of ELM Institute. *An assessment of the existing staffing patterns and personnel required in a hospice to deliver interdisciplinary patient care and the problems related to delivering humanistic care to hospice patients.* (Prepared under DHEW Contract No. HRA 232-79-0082.) Hyattsville, MD: Bureau of Health Professions, Health Resources Administration, 1980 July.

14. Wilson, English, and Research Staff.

15. English, D. J., and Wilson, D. C. The hospice concept. In: *Supplement to Delegate Manual: Association of Community Cancer Centers, 1978.* Bethesda, MD: ELM Services, Inc., revised 1979.

16. *HEW Secretary's Task Force on Hospice.* Washington, D.C.: U.S. Department of Health, Education and Welfare, Office of the Secretary, 1978 Dec.

17. Wilson, D. C. Alternative models of hospice care. In: *The "How To" of Hospice Care* (Report of the Third National Hospice Symposium). Kentfield, CA: Hospice of Marin, 1977. pp. 10-17.

18. Wilson, English, and Research Staff.

19. National Hospice Organization. *Delivery and payment.*

20. Wilson, English, and Research Staff.

21. *HEW Secretary's Task Force on Hospice.*

22. Lack, S. A. Philosophy and organization of a hospice program. In: Garfield, C. A., editor. *Psychosocial Care of the Dying Patient.* San Francisco: University of California School of Medicine, 1976.

23. National Hospice Organization. *Standards of a Hospice Program of Care,* 6th revision. McLean, VA: NHO, 1979.

24. Wilson, English, and Research Staff.

25. *HEW Secretary's Task Force on Hospice.*

26. Wilson, D. C., Ajemian, I., and Mount, B. Montreal (1975) — The Royal Victoria Hospital Palliative Care Service. In: Davidson, G. W., editor. *The Hospice — Development and Administration.* Washington, DC: Hemisphere Publishing Corporation, 1978, pp. 3-19.

27. Tehan, C. B. Hospice home care programs. In: Corr, C. A., and Corr, D. M., editors. *Hospice Care: Principles and Practice.* New York: Springer Publishing Co., 1983, pp. 281-93.

28. Grinslade, S., and Reko, R. Hospital-based inpatient hospice units: Planning considerations. In: Corr, C. A., and Corr, D. M., editors. *Hospice Care: Principles and Practice.* New York: Springer Publishing Co., 1983, pp. 294-307.

29. *Proceedings from the first national conference on hospice finance and administration. London, April 1981.* London: St. Christopher's Hospice, 1982, pp. 61-63.

30. Buckingham, R. W., and Lupu, D. A comparative study of hospice services in the United States. *American Journal of Public Health.* 1982 May. 72(5):455-63.

31. National Hospice Organization. *President's Letter.* 1982 Sept. (This newsletter contains the text of Amendment to the Social Security Act concerning

hospice reimbursement passed by Congress August 1982 as part of the Tax Equity and Fiscal Responsibility Act.)

32. English and Wilson. *Development of guidelines.*

33. English and Wilson. Steps in development of a hospice program.

34. Lack.

35. National Hospice Organization. *Standards,* 6th revision.

36. Kübler-Ross, E. *On Death and Dying.* New York: Macmillan Publishing Co., 1969.

37. Ajemian, I., and Mount, B., editors. *The Royal Victoria Hospital Manual on Palliative/Hospice Care.* New York: Arno Press, 1980.

38. Vachon, M. L. S. Motivation and stress experienced by staff working with the terminally ill. *Death Education.* 1978. 2:113-22.

39. English and Wilson. *Development of guidelines.*

40. Wilson. How to obtain community support.

41. Salladay, S. A. The administrative role in hospice planning and organization. *Death Education.* 1982. 6(3):227-48.

42. English and Wilson. Steps in development of a hospice program.

43. General Accounting Office.

44. English and Wilson. *Development of guidelines.*

45. National Hospice Organization. *Standards,* 6th revision.

46. Saunders, C. Hospice care. *American Journal of Medicine.* 1978 Nov. 65:726-28.

47. Lack.

48. National Hospice Organization. *Standards,* 6th revision.

49. Ajemian and Mount.

50. Saunders.

51. National Hospice Organization. *Standards,* 6th revision.

52. English and Wilson. *Development of guidelines.*

53. Ducanis, A. J., and Golin, A. K. *The interdisciplinary health care team.* Germantown, MD: Aspen Systems Corporation, 1979.

54. English and Wilson. *Development of guidelines.*

55. Koff.

56. Wilson, English, and Research Staff.

57. Vachon.

58. Stoddard, S. *The hospice movement: A better way of caring for the dying.* New York: Stein and Day, 1978.

59. Ajemian and Mount.

60. Vachon.

61. Beszterczey, A. Staff stress on a newly developed palliative care service. *Canadian Psychiatric Association Journal.* 1977. 22:347-53.

62. Ajemian and Mount.

63. English, D. J. Can hospice be accomplished financially? In: *Major Addresses of the Institute on Hospices, Chicago, November 16-17, 1978.* St. Louis, MO: Catholic Hospital Association, 1978.

64. Parks, P. Evaluation of hospice care is needed. *Hospitals, J.A.H.A.* 1979. 53(22):68-69.

Part 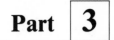 3

Public Policy Issues Related to Hospice Programs

Chapter 12

Perspectives on the Public Policy Debate

Linda H. Aiken, Ph.D.,
and Martita M. Marx, Dr.P.H.

Introduction

The public policy debate on hospice care centers on the appropriate mix of medical and supportive services for terminal cancer patients and how such services should be paid for within existing insurance programs. In this chapter, we review lessons learned from past decisions to change health care reimbursement that are applicable to the hospice debate, examine what is known about the benefits and costs of hospice care, and discuss the role of research in the formulation of social policy.

Background to the Public Policy Debate

Cancer is the most frightening of all diseases. Although not the leading cause of death or disability, cancer research ranks first in national biomedical research priorities.[1,2] The public's immense concern derives from the extended periods of suffering associated with terminal cancer and from the painful and disfiguring aspects of cancer treatment even if successful. It is not surprising, therefore, that over the past decade the debate about care of cancer patients, particularly those in the terminal stages, has captured the public's attention.

This chapter was first published in the November 1982 issue of *American Psychologist*. Copyright 1982 by the American Psychological Association. Reprinted by permission of the publisher and authors.

It is generally agreed that we need more effective and humane care for terminally ill cancer patients. But how to provide such care has become a progressively troubled national debate. At the patient care level, the debate focuses on the appropriate mix of medical interventions and psychological and family supportive care. At the public policy level, the debate concerns methods of payment that will make needed services accessible without resulting in costly duplication of services and facilities or exploitation of the dying by proprietary interests.

The current debate has evolved as a result of two developments: first, the increasing sophistication of technologies that can sustain life in situations formerly considered hopeless; second, the rapid growth of a new type of health care organization in the United States known as hospices.

The hospice movement in this country grew out of the belief that traditional medical care, with its emphasis on curative medicine and the technological imperative, had become increasingly inhumane and insensitive to the needs of dying people and their families.[3] Many have come to feel that curative technology and life support systems are being inappropriately used in the care of terminal cancer patients, resulting in the prolongation of suffering and physical life without regard for its quality. Moreover, many feel that such care, which usually requires hospitalization, isolates the dying from family and friends at the very time when they are most needed.[4,5].

In the early 1970s, physicians and other health professionals, particularly those in hospitals, showed little interest in accommodating the special needs of cancer patients who did not want to undergo painful treatment when the prognosis looked hopeless, but who instead wanted relief from symptoms for as long as possible and an opportunity to die with dignity near loved ones. As a result, proponents of what became known as hospice care established alternative care programs either as freestanding community organizations or as separate units in hospitals with autonomous medical and nursing staff. That it captured much popular interest is evident from the very rapid growth that has occurred since the establishment in 1974 of the first U.S. hospice in New Haven, Connecticut, modeled after St. Christopher's Hospice in London. By 1981, the Joint Commission on Accreditation of Hospitals (JCAH) had identified 800 hospice programs, 51 percent having become operational after January 1980.[6]

The rapid growth of hospices has created a vocal new constituency for the enactment of special provisions to pay for hospice services under existing public insurance programs, particularly Medicare. Public response to improving services for the terminally ill has been overwhelmingly positive. However, many physicians fear that patients and families will not really be better off in hospices. Instead, they may be isolated from medical care needed to control the disease process and thereby suffer more than necessary. The primary debate about hospice care focuses on whether terminally ill people and their families can be better cared for in terms of comfort and quality of life if care is provided in their homes or in special institutions as opposed to conventional inpatient institutional medical care.

A secondary issue in the hospice debate concerns the comparative costs of hospice care. Advocates for hospices argue that significant cost savings can be achieved by substituting supportive services in the home or hospice for hospital care. The cost savings potential of hospices adds significantly to their appeal.

There is increasing concern about the high cost of dying in this country, especially now that so many health and social programs are targets for budget reductions. Medicare, for example, will spend almost $50 billion in 1982, accounting for one out of every $15 spent by the federal government.[7] Sixty-five percent of those who died in 1976 were Medicare beneficiaries. Although they represented only 6.4 percent of all Medicare enrollees, they accounted for 31 percent of total Medicare payments.[8] Obviously, the nation does not want to economize at the expense of the terminally ill. However, if there is evidence that hospice care is both better and less costly, there is even more reason to try to make such care readily available.

The cost-savings potential of hospices has not been demonstrated to everyone's satisfaction. Some analysts remain worried about encouraging the growth of a new health care institution that may add to the public's expense at a time when we are faced with reducing present commitments for basic health services for the poor and the elderly, including reductions in essential services such as immunizations and prenatal care for pregnant women.

This chapter examines the hospice debate within the larger context of health policy. First, we review lessons learned from some of the nation's past decisions to change health care reimbursement that seem to be applicable to the hospice debate. Second, we examine what is known to date about the benefits and costs of hospice care. Finally, we conclude with a discussion of the role of research in public policy formulation.

Unanticipated Consequences of Modifying Payment for Health Services

Over the years, there have been many proposals for reorganizing the financing of health services in this country to provide universal health insurance coverage. Instead, the nation has pursued an incremental policy of providing increased public subsidies to certain categories of people, sometimes determined by age group, sometimes by income levels, and sometimes by disease categories. Although incremental change is usually expedient in the short run, the long-term consequences are often unanticipated and contrary to what was intended.

In reviewing the consequences of major changes in reimbursement for health services over the past 30 years, a number of generalizations can be made:

1. New benefits stimulate greater demand for services than originally anticipated.
2. Once a new benefit is offered, new categories of patients not originally considered to need it suddenly acquire it as a right.
3. Cost savings achieved by substituting new services for more expensive alternatives for some patients are usually more than offset by the supplemental use of new services by others.
4. Publicly supported services replace those previously provided by family members or volunteers.
5. Reimbursing services results in a shift toward more expensive professional caregivers.
6. New benefits encourage the growth of new organizations and interest groups that over time change the nature and costs of the new services.
7. New benefits can encourage the emergence of new provider organizations with different social commitments, quality standards, and operating arrangements than those anticipated or intended.
8. The cost-savings potential of technology is usually overestimated.
9. Fee-for-service payment encourages the provision of those services for which reimbursement policies are most generous irrespective of the needs of patients.

Most previous modifications in policies regarding payment for health services have resulted in greater than predicted costs and, in some cases, care that was less than the desired quality. The following examples are discussed to gain a better understanding of the lessons learned that might be applicable to the hospice policy debate.

Nursing Homes

Nursing homes developed largely as a byproduct of social welfare legislation, beginning with the Social Security Act of 1935.[9] Its major impetus was to provide poor elderly with sufficient income to support themselves and allow public almshouses to be closed. But pensions, it turned out, were not a substitute for institutional care for the elderly who were infirm as well as poor, and it became impossible to close public institutions.

Some elderly chose to use their new cash benefits to purchase services in sheltered institutional settings. However, the demand for institutional care created by the new benefit far outstripped the available capacity of religious and not-for-profit, voluntary community facilties. Proprietary homes filled the void and became the dominant providers of care. Thus, legislation designed to phase out substandard institutions actually served to accelerate the growth of proprietary interest. Care of the elderly became a profitable business, managed by groups with different social values, standards of quality, and organizational arrangements than had originally been anticipated.

Although the die was cast for nursing homes in this early legislation, the passage of Medicare and Medicaid in 1965 further contributed to the national problem by failing to address nursing homes directly. Most coverage of nursing home services was rejected outright by the designers of Medicare, but almost by default, skilled nursing care came to be designated as a reimbursable service under Medicaid, and even patients who entered nursing homes with their own means became eligible after exhausting all their available funds. Once there were tens of thousands of people in nursing homes, there was no way to discontinue paying for their care, despite the low standards that often prevailed.

In an effort to contain costs in this large and ballooning industry, the cost-reimbursement method used for paying for hospital care was cast aside, and daily rates were instituted instead. Although then expedient, daily rates that do not vary for patients with substantially differing care needs have resulted in the development of perverse financial incentives for nursing home operators. Existing incentives discourage discharge of patients capable of caring for themselves and paradoxically discourage the admission of those most in need of skilled nursing care. The end result is a large number of inappropriately institutionalized, publicly subsidized patients in nursing homes and a significant backlog of patients requiring nursing care waiting for nursing home placement in expensive, acute-care hospitals.

It is frequently said that if we are to avoid the same mistakes in hospice reimbursement, the lessons learned from nursing homes should be studied carefully.

End-Stage Renal Disease Program

Also of relevance to the hospice debate is the nation's decade of experience following the 1972 Social Security amendment extending Medicare coverage to practically all Americans with end-stage renal disease (ESRD). The intent of that legislation was similar to hospice in that its primary purpose was to improve access to services. Further, it covers patients with a specific categorical disease, just as hospices are primarily concerned currently with cancer patients. The ESRD program, like hospices, was only secondarily concerned with the costs of care; that is, could end-stage renal disease be as effectively treated using less expensive modes of care?

Again, a persistent underestimation of total costs has characterized the ESRD program since its inception. The sponsor of the bill in the Senate projected that the amendment would eventually cost $90 to $110 million a year, "a minor cost to maintain life."[10] Projected costs in 1980 were $1.4 billion and were expected to rise to $4.6 billion by 1995.[11]

Three unanticipated factors contributed to the higher than expected costs. First, the number of beneficiaries of the new program was underestimated. The program was originally intended to provide lifesaving care to people in the prime of life, but once benefits were available, an increased number of the elderly used them. At the inception of the program, only 5 percent of ESRD patients were over 65 years of age; by 1978, one-fifth were over 65.[12] Some worry about similar consequences for hospices. Once provided for terminal cancer patients, will entirely different categories of patients claim a right to similar services?

Second, the anticipated use of less costly home dialysis did not occur. At the program's inception, 40 percent of patients were maintained on home dialysis, but this dropped steadily to 15 percent by 1978. The reimbursement regulations unfortunately contained a number of financial disincentives for patients to remain on home dialysis. Out-of-pocket costs to patients were significantly less if dialysis occurred in institutional settings. Most hospitals, however, were not organized to provide long-term dialysis for outpatients. As in the case of nursing homes, proprietary interests again entered the void and now provide 40 percent of the hemodialysis.[13]

Third, the cost-savings potential of kidney transplantation has, to date, been vastly overestimated. Transplants have not had the long-term effectiveness originally anticipated. Patients often require multiple transplants, and many never receive transplants at all, which has resulted in an ever increasing number of people depending on lifelong dialysis. An Institute of Medicine[14] committee anticipated many of these problems as early as the first year of the program and unanimously concluded that coverage of discrete categories of diseases would be an inappropriate course to follow in the future. Many see special hospice reimbursement as another attempt to provide categorical insurance coverage, a strategy that has been problematic in the past.

Substitution of Ambulatory Services for Institutional Care

A last illustration that should give us pause has been the overall experience with expansion of ambulatory care services. Over the past decade there have been a number of attempts to confirm the logical assumption that comprehensive ambulatory care will reduce the need for expensive hospitalization. However, except in such closed systems as health maintenance organizations (HMOs) where the fee-for-service incentive has been removed, overall costs rise due to increased utilization of ambulatory services without much accompanying change in hospitalization.[15] Ambulatory services generally supplement rather than substitute for hospital services.

This has also been the case for most programs for the elderly that have tried to substitute community-based alternatives such as adult day care and homemaker services for nursing home and hospital care. A major problem plaguing these efforts, which could emerge as an issue in hospice care, is that community-based programs generally increase total costs by increasing overall health service consumption by patients who are not likely to use significant inpatient services even in the absence of community programs.

A recent controlled experiment evaluating the costs and effects of adult day care and homemaker services found that overall costs were significantly higher for people having access to the community services.[16,17] Most patients used day care and homemaker services *in addition to* hospital and nursing home care. Moreover, those using the community services were not the group at high risk of long hospital and nursing home stays, so the services did not substitute for inpatient care.

An additional problem faced in home care or community services is that publicly supported services tend to replace those currently provided by families or volunteers, a serious concern in relation to hospice care. A recent study by the General Accounting Office[18] of Medicare home health services concluded that publicly financed aide services supplant support by family and friends 28 percent of the time. Of further concern to the GAO was the difficulty of ascertaining which patients really needed services in the home. These concerns derive from a 336 percent increase in Medicare home health care expenditures from 1976 to 1981. The number of Medicare enrollees using home health care almost doubled between 1974 and 1978, and the number of visits per person serviced also increased. In 1978, 12 percent of the users of home health services accounted for almost half of the visits; 25,000 users in this group received an average of 135 visits that year. The difficulty experienced to date in estimating use of currently covered Medicare home health services raises serious doubts as to whether there is much basis for estimating the costs of extending special home care benefits to the dying under new hospice legislation.

A variety of home services are now being provided by profit-making businesses. Expenditures for proprietary-sponsored home care in 1979 were estimated to be close to $3 billion.[19] As Medicare and private insurance companies broaden home health benefits, proprietary interests can also be expected to expand.

As a general rule, for every inpatient admission actually avoided by new ambulatory services, several new cases are drawn into the health care system by virtue of more accessible outpatient care. There is also the risk of replacing volunteer services with publicly financed care. This is not to say that community care programs or outpatient services that do not avoid institutionalization or result in cost savings are not important. Clearly such services often result in better care — an appropriate and legitimate purpose for developing such programs. But accurate anticipation of likely consequences needs careful consideration in the current hospice discussions.

The Hospice Policy Debate

It is often suggested that health professionals give insufficient concern to quality of life of the sick and disabled and unnecessarily overmedicalize the natural events of life — birth, old age, and death. Hospitals, nursing homes, and health professionals have all been openly criticized for their failures to provide sensitive and empathetic medical care and for the excessive use of technology. In response, women's groups have promoted the development of small birthing centers or nurse-midwife-assisted home deliveries for uncomplicated births.[20,21] Noninstitutional community settings have been sought to provide more humane care for the elderly.[22] Hospices are a model for providing a supportive environment for death at home or in special homelike settings with dignity and minimal professional "interference."

Hospice Care

The hospice movement has focused on alternatives for the care of terminally ill cancer patients, who make up about 95 percent of all hospice patients. Such care is directed toward patients who no longer have a reasonable chance of cure or remission. Hospices try to admit patients who have six months or less to live. The average length of stay is about 47 days.[23] Usually to be eligible for hospice care, patients must have a family member or friend who provides continuing involvement.

There is considerable variation among hospices in the services provided, but there are some core elements. Nursing care is central. Almost all provide home nursing care, and some have inpatient facilities as well. Ideally, nurses are available 24 hours a day, but this varies. The dominant objective of care is comfort, both physical and psychological, for both the patient and the family. When appropriate, patients are cared for in their own homes. Heroic measures are not used to prolong life, and death is treated as a natural phenomenon to be discussed openly among family members.

Some hospices provide other support services. They include: homemaker or home health aides, physician home visits or transportation to the physician, social and psychological counseling, procurement of special equipment needed in home care, and respite care and bereavement counseling for the family.

Hospices have developed innovative methods for treating chronic pain. The concern about narcotic addiction, so prevalent in acute hospital settings, is deemphasized. Instead, pain is controlled by potent oral analgesic mixtures and sometimes by unconventional drugs such as marijuana. The goal is to control pain but to maintain as much alertness as possible.

Most of the controversy surrounding hospice treatment concerns when patients should be designated as terminal, and once the terminal prognosis is made, how aggressive the treatment should be. Many physicians, patients, and families wish to go on fighting for life to the very end, and hospitals and clinical research settings are prepared to offer that level of care.[24] Some patients and families prefer to know when there is no hope for cure so that other alternatives can be considered. However, physicians are reluctant to predict length of survival. Yates, McKegney, and Kun[25] found that physicians' predictions of prognosis were relatively inaccurate, with actual survival plus or minus one month coinciding with that predicted in only 16 percent of patients. Except inpatients who were very ill and had short prognoses of three to four months, survival was consistently underestimated. On the one hand, referral of patients into hospice programs too early might not be in their best interest and might deprive them of medical intervention that could slow the disease process. On the other, the reluctance of physicians to make a prognosis serves to deny patients the opportunity to choose hospice services.

Symptom control has been the source of considerable debate among hospice advocates and between hospice and conventional care physicians. Some hospice proponents advocate withdrawal of active treatment and the provision of psychological support and palliative care until death. Many oncologists, and hospice proponents as well, believe that dying people have reversible medical problems that should be actively treated by radiation therapy, surgery, and other techniques aimed at symptom relief, not cure.[26,27] Sylvia Lack, the medical director of the New Haven hospice who came to the United States from St. Christopher's Hospice in London, fears that patients cared for at home in this country will become isolated from effective medical care and suffer unnecessarily from vomiting, pain, and other controllable symptoms.

> There is far too much talk in death and dying circles in this country about psychological and emotional problems, and far too little about making patients comfortable. Discomfort looms large in the lives of patients with terminal illness. Without pain, well nursed, with bowels controlled, clean mouths, and a caring friend available, psychological problems fall into manageable perspective.[28]

The debate about the best method to care for terminal cancer has gone on in medical circles for years. Public attention has increased from efforts of hospice advocates to change legislation governing public insurance policies and achieve more favorable financing for hospice services.

Ultimately, the continued growth of new noninstitutional health programs requires change in the structure of health insurance. Our insurance system largely pays for institutional care, discouraging patients from seeking care in community or home settings, however appropriate to their needs, because they are not reimbursed. Hospices are like many other efforts to expand community-based care, such as community mental health services, nurse-midwifery and birth centers, and community-based care for the elderly.

The answers to two deceptively simple questions are required to provide a rationale for changing reimbursement for services to the terminally ill:

1. Is the impact of hospice care on the quality of life of the terminally ill and their families as good as or better than conventional arrangements?
2. If the quality of life of hospice patients is the same or better than that of patients under conventional care, would there be a major change in the cost to insurers of adding a new hospice benefit?

Quality of Life

Quality of life for the terminally ill seems to have two major dimensions: self-perceptions of general well-being and feelings of discomfort. Yates and his colleagues[29] at the Vermont Regional Cancer Center have identified the factors important to patients' assessment of well-being and discomfort. Perceptions of well-being relate primarily to independence in self-care, desire for food, and overall assessment of condition. Discomfort is evaluated in large part by pain and difficulty in sleeping.

The hospice movement gives special attention to each of these factors. The emphasis on home care promotes independence in self-care that is difficult to achieve in hospital settings. The efforts of hospices to "demedicalize" the dying process may promote a more positive outlook and avoid some of the iatrogenic side effects of invasive procedures routinely carried out in hospitals, such as blood tests and intravenous fluids. Symptom control is a major objective of hospice care, and the available literature indicates that some hospices have developed successful strategies to control pain.[30,31]

Studies of the care of terminal cancer patients in hospitals point to a number of serious problems related to maintaining quality of life. Freeman[32] evaluated the extent to which terminal patients in hospitals received relief of symptoms and the use of least noxious but effective treatments. His findings are startling. "Less-than-optimal" treatment was given to 92 percent of terminal patients for pain, 91 percent for nausea and vomiting, 100 percent suffering from breathing problems, and 93 percent for pulmonary secretions. Almost all patients received routine, slightly noxious, unnecessary procedures such as monitoring vital signs at midnight. Twenty-seven percent were in restraints, and 43 percent were turned frequently in spite of pain.

Despite studies of the negative consequences of hospitalization and the positive aspects of hospice care, the actual differences in the quality of life are uncertain. Physicians and hospital staffs have been influenced by the ideology of the hospice movement and have incorporated many aspects of hospice care into mainstream medical practice. The hospice movement has succeeded, to some extent, in humanizing care for the dying in hospitals. Also, there is considerable variation among hospices, and differences in the quality of life of hospice patients might be expected to vary accordingly.

There are three major organizational arrangements for hospice services: hospital-sponsored, freestanding, and home health agency-sponsored. These three types of hospices differ significantly in extent of physician involvement, central control over inpatient and home care services, the use of inpatient care, the use of medical interventions, and the scope of social and psychological support services offered.[33]

The hospice movement has placed greater importance on the quality of life of family members than has usually been the case in conventional medical practice. Such services are not conventionally covered under insurance. To provide a rationale for extending coverage to families, it is important to know whether families benefit from hospice services. Bereavement counseling is a central service of hospice care but one of uncertain effectiveness. The increased vulnerability to illness of survivors following the death of a family member is well documented. Significant increases in mortality, alcoholism and drug abuse, reactive depression, and inability to work have been reported among survivors in the year or more following death of a family member.[34-37]

Although an array of preventive care services has been provided for survivors, rarely has effectiveness been carefully evaluated.[38] Only three such studies were found in a review of the literature; two indicated that survivors fare better after bereavement counseling,[39,40] and one found no effect.[41] Positive outcomes included fewer physical symptoms, fewer physician visits, fewer cases of marked depression, less dependence on alcohol and drugs, and greater capacity to work for families receiving such services. But given the inconsistent findings of the few available evaluations, caution seems warranted until further research confirms the effectiveness of bereavement counseling.

Judgments about quality of life necessarily involve human values. Some terminally ill cancer patients and their families want to try every treatment available to extend life. They are willing to sacrifice comfort for the chance of cure or remission.[42] Others prefer to live their remaining days as normally as possible with minimal medical interference but with access to services when needed. The hospice debate is about choices. Insurance now offers families the first option—pursuit of every possible treatment. Hospice proponents believe families should have the opportunity to make other choices without financial penalty and with the assurance that medical help will be there when they need it. If the latter criterion (access to needed medical services) is met, the only remaining question relates to the additional cost of hospice care.

Cost of Hospice Care

If hospice care proves to be the same as or more effective than conventional care in maintaining the quality of life of the terminally ill and their families, the costs would have to be staggering to be seen as relevant in the debate. Two types of information, however, are needed on the comparative costs of hospice care: (a) the additional costs, if any, of hospice care over and above current expenditures in the last year of life for care of terminally ill cancer patients treated in conventional settings, and (b) an estimate of the frequency with which the new benefit might be used.

Cost savings from hospice care are likely to depend on the ability of hospices to reduce inpatient hospital care. The more intensive the home services provided, the more days of hospitalization would have to be avoided to offset the costs of home care. In addition, the cost-savings potential of hospices could be compromised if volunteer and family services are replaced by paid professional care.

Several small studies suggest cost savings. Bloom and Kissick[43] studied the billed charges of the last two weeks of life for a matched group of cancer patients cared for at home and in hospitals. The cost was over 10 times greater for hospitalized patients. The California Department of Health Services[44] compared the cost of hospice care in four programs with hospital care for terminally ill patients and identified "potential" net savings of over $2,000 per person. The major limitation of these studies and all others to date is that the time frame is not sufficient to evaluate differences in total costs of care in the last year of life. It is not clear whether patients have already incurred large costs before admission to hospices, and therefore use hospice services in addition to considerable conventional medical care in the last year of life, or whether the "potential" savings are real reductions in total costs.

The costs of hospice care vary significantly among hospices. The National Cancer Institute[45] study of comparative costs of hospice care found substantial variance among the three institutions studied, all partially or fully supported by public funds. The average cost of a home visit varied from $60.57 to $91.37, and the cost per inpatient day (inpatient hospice beds) ranged from $143.44 to $249.92.

Three factors are likely to be important in predicting the eventual use of a new hospice benefit. First, reductions in families' out-of-pocket expenses for hospice care should increase the number of patients electing the new benefit. Second, the attitudes of physicians about referring patients to hospices, and the acceptance by families of hospice care, will also affect the proportion of terminally ill patients likely to use the benefit. Third, new categories of patients may claim a right to hospicelike services once they are reimbursed for the terminally ill. Close to 400,000 Americans died from cancer in 1977.[46] Cancer deaths are expected to rise to 467,000 by the year 2000. There are few other diseases where predictions of survival can be made in weeks or months. But there are many people in need of expanded home health services, and once covered by insurance for the terminally ill, they may have to be provided on a broader scale.

All treatments for cancer patients are subjected to rigorous laboratory tests and clinical trials before they are made available for general use. Testimony from advocates of laetrile and a few families who believed in its effectiveness was not sufficient to warrant its widespread dissemination in the absence of research evidence of its effectiveness. Yet, in the case of hospices, a new form of care for cancer patients has been introduced, and the groups involved advocate that it be paid for and expanded without an objective clinical evaluation. The effectiveness and costs of new services, like new drugs, can be independently assessed by research in a manner acceptable to experts in the field of cancer. Proposals to change the payment system for services for the terminally ill led the Robert Wood Johnson Foundation and the John A. Hartford Foundation to join with the Health Care Financing Administration to support a national demonstration and study of hospice care.

The National Hospice Study, directed by David S. Greer and his associate Vincent Mor at the School of Medicine, Brown University, was launched in 1980. Twenty-six hospices from 16 states were chosen from among 236 applicants to receive Medicare, and in some cases Medicaid, waivers for a two-year period. The waivers provide payment for hospice services excluded under existing reimbursement policies. Hospices receiving waivers fall into three categories: hospital-sponsored, home health agency-sponsored, and freestanding. All provide home care, and some also provide inpatient care. They vary on other dimensions, including the nature of medical supervision, linkages with hospitals, the range of social, psychological, and other support services offered, composition of staff, use of volunteers, and number of patients served. Fourteen similar hospices are participating in the study but do not receive reimbursement waivers, which will provide an opportunity to evaluate the effects of expanded reimbursement on scope of services, costs to patients, and cost to insurers.

In-home data collection over five to six points in time will be undertaken to study the quality of life of patients and families cared for in hospices with reimbursement waivers, those without waivers, and a matched comparison group of terminal cancer patients receiving care within conventional medical arrangements. The impact of hospice and conventional care on quality of life and social and psychological costs to family members will be documented during the terminal phase of illness and continue at least three months after the patient's death. The sample size of hospice and conventional care patients will be large enough to permit patients to be matched on all relevant factors, including age, sex, type of cancer, and functional status and severity of illness.

Total costs of medical care will be estimated for both hospice and conventional patients. Families are maintaining medical cost diaries to record reimbursed and out-of-pocket expenditures, and insurance and institutional records will also be audited.

Discussion

Hospice proponents convey a sense of urgency about the need for a new policy on reimbursement for hospice care. But terminal illness is neither a new nor short-run problem for social policy. Cancer is responsible for a larger proportion of deaths than ever before. Good public policy must plan for the long range and not respond only to immediate concerns and political pressures. Thus, it would be unfortunate not to make full use of available data and experience, not only to ensure a sensitive response to the needs of the terminally ill and their families but also to develop policies consistent with the nation's overall objectives in health maintenance and medical care provision.

Professional opinion, special interests, politics, and values will all play some role in decisions about hospices. As this debate proceeds, it is useful to keep in mind that health services and medical care of known value are being reduced or eliminated from public programs in response to economic constraints. In this context, it is even more compelling to ensure that new services covered are efficacious and justify their costs.

References

1. Rice, D. P., Feldman, J. J., and White, K. L. *The Current Burden of Illness in the United States.* Washington, DC: National Academy of Sciences, Institute of Medicine, 1976.

2. Strickland, S. P. *Politics, Science, and Dread Disease.* Cambridge, MA: Harvard University Press, 1972.

3. Stoddard, S. *The Hospice Movement: A Better Way of Caring for the Dying.* New York: Vintage, 1974.

4. Cohen, K. P. *Hospice: Prescription for Terminal Care.* Germantown, MD: Aspen Systems Corporation, 1979.

5. Koff, T. H. *Hospice: A Caring Community.* Cambridge, MA: Winthrop Publishers, Inc., 1980.

6. Falknor, H. P., and Kugler, D. JCAH hospice project, interim report: Phase I. Mimeo, Joint Commission on Accreditation of Hospitals, Chicago, 1981 July.

7. Davis, K. Medicare reconsidered. Paper presented at the Duke University Private Sector Conference on the Financial Support of Health Care of the Elderly and the Indigent, Durham, North Carolina, 1982 Mar.

8. Lubitz, J., Gornick, M., and Prihoda, R. *Use and Costs of Medicare Services in the Last Year of Life.* Washington, DC: U.S. Department of Health and Human Services, Health Care Financing Administration, 1981.

9. Vladeck, B. C. *Unloving Care: The Nursing Home Tragedy.* New York: Basic Books, 1980.

10. Congressional Record, 1972. 118, 33004.

11. Rettig, R. A. The politics of health cost containment: End-stage renal disease. *Bulletin of the New York Academy of Medicine.* 1980. 56:115-38.

12. Rettig.

13. Relman, A. S. The new medical-industrial complex. *New England Journal of Medicine.* 1980. 303:963-70.

14. Institute of Medicine. *Disease by Disease: Toward National Health Insurance?* Washington, DC: National Academy of Sciences, 1973.

15. Lewis, C. E., and Keairnes, H. W. Controlling costs of medical care by expanding insurance coverage. *New England Journal of Medicine.* 1970. 282:1405-12.

16. Weissert, W. G., Wan, T. T., and others. Cost-effectiveness of day care services for the chronically ill: A randomized experiment. *Medical Care.* 1980. 18:567-84.

17. Weissert, G.W., Wan, T. T., and others. Cost-effectiveness of homemaker services for the chronically ill: A randomized experiment. *Inquiry.* 1980. 17(3):230-43.

18. General Accounting Office. *Medicare Home Health Services: A Difficult Program to Control* (HRD-81-155). Washington, DC: GAO, 1981.

19. Relman.

20. Arms, S. *Immaculate Deception—A New Look at Women and Childbirth in America.* Boston: Houghton Mifflin, 1975.

21. Corea, G. *The Hidden Malpractice: How American Medicine Mistreats Women.* New York: Harcourt Brace Jovanovich, 1977.

22. Vladeck.

23. Buckingham, R. W., and Lupu, D. A comparative study of hospice services in the United States. *American Journal of Public Health.* 1982 May. 72(5):455-63.

24. Krant, M. J. The hospice movement. *New England Journal of Medicine.* 1978. 299:546-49.

25. Yates, J. W., McKegney, F. P., and Kun, L. E. A comparative study of home nursing care of patients with advanced cancer. In: *Proceedings of the American Cancer Society, 3rd National Conference on Human Values of Cancer.* New York: American Cancer Society, 1982.

26. Yates, McKegney, and Kun.

27. Potter, J. F. A challenge for the hospice movement. *New England Journal of Medicine.* 1980. 302:53-55.

28. Lack, S. A. Characteristics of a hospice program of care. In: Davidson, G. W., editor. *The Hospice: Development and Administration.* Washington, DC: Hemisphere Publishing Corporation, 1978.

29. Yates, McKegney, and Kun.

30. Koff.

31. Lack.

32. Freeman, W. L. An audit of hospital care for terminal cancer patients. Paper presented at the meeting of the Robert Wood Johnson Clinical Scholars Program, Scottsdale, Arizona, 1980 Nov.

33. Buckingham and Lupu.

34. Helsing, K. J., and Szklo, M. Mortality after bereavement. *American Journal of Epidemiology.* 1981 July. 114(1):41-52.

35. Klerman, G. L., and Izen, J. E. The effects of bereavement and grief on physical health and general well-being. In: Reichsman, R., editor. *Advances in Psychosomatic Medicine: Epidemiological Studies in Psychosomatic Medicine.* Basel, Switzerland: Karger, 1975.

36. Rahe, R. H. The pathway between subjects' recent life changes and their near-future illness reports. In: Dohrenwend, B. S., and Dohrenwend, B. P., editors. *Stressful Life Events: Their Nature and Effects.* New York: Wiley, 1974.

37. Rees, W. D., and Lutkins, S. G. Mortality of bereavement. *British Medical Journal.* 1967. 4:13-16.

38. Parkes, C. M. Bereavement counselling: Does it work? *British Medical Journal.* 1980. 281:3-6.

39. Gerber, I., Weiner, A., and others. Brief therapy to the aged bereaved. In: Schoenberg, B., and Gerber, I., editors. *Bereavement: Its Psychological Aspects.* New York: Columbia University Press, 1975.

40. Raphael, B. Preventive intervention with the recently bereaved. *Archives of General Psychiatry.* 1977. 34:1450-54.

41. Polak, P. R., Egan, D., and others. Prevention in mental health: A controlled study. *American Journal of Psychiatry.* 1975. 132:146-49.

42. Krakoff, I. H. The case for patients with advanced cancer: Not everyone needs a hospice. *CA—A Cancer Journal.* 1979. 29:108-11.

43. Bloom, B. S., and Kissick, P. D. Home and hospital cost of terminal illness. *Medical Care.* 1980. 18:560-64.

44. California Department of Health Services. Palliative care service pilot project. Report to the 1980 California legislature on the hospice project, pursuant to Assembly Bill 1586, CH 1324, 1978, Sacramento, 1980.

45. Kay, L. L., Cummings, M. A., and Mundell, M. B. Hospice: A cost analysis of three programs. Kaiser-Permanente Medical Care Program, Southern California Region. Funded by National Cancer Institute, Contract No. 85375, 1981 July.

46. General Accounting Office. *Report to the Congress: Hospice Care—A Growing Concept in the United States* (HRD-79-50). Washington, DC: U.S. Government Printing Office, 1979.